Praise for

THE MINDFUL WAY THROUGH STRESS

"Alidina has written a very practical and engaging guide to stress reduction! Extracting much of the essence of the well-known and researched mindfulness-based stress reduction (MBSR) program, he shows how to begin practicing and experiencing the benefits of mindfulness. For those who don't have the opportunity (or time) to take the full program in person, following the wisdom of this fun-to-read guide can jump-start the integration of mindfulness into today's hectic and fast-paced lifestyles. Do yourself a favor and pause to really take in the message of this book and make room in your day to practice what is taught, and you'll definitely be glad you did."
—*Steven D. Hickman, PsyD, Executive Director, Center for Mindfulness, University of California, San Diego*

"Do you want to learn mindfulness without leaving home? If so, this is an ideal place to start. Written in an exceptionally clear and encouraging style, it is chock-full of practical wisdom, supportive research, and opportunities for self-reflection. Alidina creatively presents the gold standard of mindfulness training: MBSR. Included is a mini-course for those with little time, as well as downloadable meditations. This book is a welcome companion for anyone wishing to lead a more stress-free life."
—*Christopher K. Germer, PhD, author of* The Mindful Path to Self-Compassion

"Drawing on decades of experience with the highly successful MBSR program, this clear, practical, step-by-step guide can help anyone use mindfulness practices to feel less stressed—even in difficult circumstances."
—*Ronald D. Siegel, PsyD, author of* The Mindfulness Solution

"Everyone deserves to reduce stress—not only will you feel better, but you'll also be surprised by how MBSR unleashes your creativity and productivity. Shamash is a wonderful teacher."
—*Chade-Meng Tan, Jolly Good Fellow of Google and author of* Search Inside Yourself

"Internationally recognized mindfulness teacher and writer Shamash Alidina has written a wonderfully practical, easy-to-read book helping us to recognize the many different elements of stress and how to cope. Full of examples and step-by-step guidance, this book offers a clear path to a calmer mind and life. A gift of wisdom to help us in our busy and stressful lives."
—*Paul Gilbert, PhD, FBPsS, OBE, Head, Mental Health Research Unit, University of Derby, United Kingdom*

THE MINDFUL WAY THROUGH STRESS

THE MINDFUL WAY THROUGH STRESS

The Proven 8-Week Path to Health, Happiness, and Well-Being

SHAMASH ALIDINA

THE GUILFORD PRESS

New York   London

Published by The Guilford Press
A Division of Guilford Publications, Inc.
370 Seventh Avenue, Suite 1200, New York, NY 10001
www.guilford.com

Printed in the United States of America

This book is printed on acid-free paper.

Last digit is print number: 9   8   7   6   5   4   3   2

Library of Congress Cataloging-in-Publication Data

Alidina, Shamash.
    The mindful way through stress : the proven 8-week path to health, happiness, and well-being / Shamash Alidina.
        pages   cm
    Includes bibliographical references and index.
    ISBN 978-1-4625-0940-9 (paperback) — ISBN 978-1-4625-1793-0 (hardcover)
    1. Stress management.   2. Meditation—Therapeutic use.   3. Health.
I. Title.
    RA785.A43 2015
    613—dc23

                            2014032834

Illustrations by Christopher Reinke

This book is dedicated to all those suffering from stress. May you discover the freedom and joy of living mindfully in the present moment.

Acknowledgments

WRITING IS a great privilege. Your willingness to purchase this book helps to support me. I'd like to thank you personally for that.

I would like to thank Jon Kabat-Zinn, Saki Santorelli, and their colleagues at the Center for Mindfulness in Massachusetts for originally developing the mindfulness-based stress reduction (MBSR) program upon which this book is based. I'd particularly like to thank them for the training they've offered many others, including me. Without their team's hard work, this book wouldn't exist. I'm also grateful for the teachers at the Centre for Mindfulness Research and Practice at Bangor University, United Kingdom. Additionally, many hundreds of researchers have worked tirelessly to build the evidence base of the program, and I'm grateful for their work.

I'd like to thank all my friends and family for their kindness and support. I'm especially grateful for their readiness to put up with my silly jokes and frequent absence while writing. I'd probably be stressed out without them!

I'd like to give a big thank you to Kitty Moore and Chris Benton of the fantastic Guilford Press. They really make a wonderful team and have played a massive part in producing this book, as well as making mindfulness more accessible through many other publications. I'd like to thank Kitty for her trust in me, her guidance, and for our wonderful meetings in San Francisco. And thanks to Chris for her meticulous eye for detail, many hours of editing the manuscript, and her sound advice. I'm forever grateful for their wisdom and compassion.

I'm also aware of the many other people working behind the scenes at Guilford to produce this book. I'd like to acknowledge and thank the part they've played to develop this work.

And last, but not least, I'd like to thank Christopher Reinke for all the illustrations in this book. I'm immensely grateful for his generosity and patience with the many high-quality drawings he produced. Thank you.

Contents

Purchasers can download audio files and select practical
tools from this book at *www.guilford.com/alidina-materials.*

Introduction

SARAH WAS a typical busy working mom. Her first marriage didn't work out the way she had hoped. After the divorce, she couldn't face looking for someone else on top of everything else she had to do. She was assistant manager at a small hotel and had a 6-year-old son to look after on her own. He was a lovely boy, but certainly a handful. Teachers often called her in to discuss his aggressive behavior toward the other children. She also had to juggle helping her mother, who lived 2 hours away. If she didn't make that trip every Sunday, she was filled with pangs of guilt. Her father had died last year, and her mother was feeling terribly lonely. Sarah didn't really have time to process the emotions of losing her father, and she continued to find herself crying out of the blue.

But these were just the external pressures. Internally, she had to deal with the challenges of feeling frustrated and angry at her boss, constantly worrying about her little boy and whether he was going to be okay, and feeling sad about how life seemed so difficult at the moment.

Sarah felt like she hadn't slept well for months. She felt tired all the time, and life seemed like an enormous struggle. She couldn't see a way out of this negative cycle. She tried exercising more, but that didn't seem to help much. Then she started to have stomach pains. After a checkup, her doctor said he thought they might be due to stress. Sarah was skeptical that a physical pain could be caused by stress, and she was even more doubtful when the doctor recommended a mindfulness class. How could that possibly eliminate all the problems she was wrestling with?

Still, she didn't have any other ideas, so she decided to try it. At first she thought the classes were doing more harm than good. She couldn't relax in the class and in fact started noticing just how negative her thoughts were, which made her feel even worse. She had to admit it was nice meeting some different people, though, so she decided to take it one class at a time and keep going as long as "one more class" sounded bearable. She did the mindfulness homework, or "experiments" as the teacher called them, and gradually she began to feel different.

The real breakthrough came to Sarah in the third week, when the instructor was guiding one of the meditations. She realized that her stomach pain had almost disappeared. And more than that, she felt like she was regaining some control in her life, even though the outer circumstances hadn't changed. The following week she was far more aware of the thoughts that popped up in her mind, and they didn't get hold of her like they used to. Her sleep improved, and she learned new ways to deal with her difficult emotions in the weeks that followed. By the end of the course, she felt like she had learned not just a set of techniques but a way of living—*mindful living*—that seemed life saving in some ways.

Is This Book for You?

Sarah's story is not a fantasy; these are the kinds of results that thousands of people all over the world are finding from practicing mindfulness. Mounting scientific evidence from hundreds of universities—including dedicated centers at the University of Massachusetts Medical School in the United States and the University of Oxford in the United Kingdom—strongly suggests that mindfulness not only reduces stress but also gently builds an inner strength so that future stressors have less impact on our happiness and physical well-being.

By reading this book and practicing the exercises, you will learn approaches that are ancient yet profoundly beneficial in our modern world. Even brain scans have revealed helpful changes taking place in just 8 weeks of regular practice—a program that is outlined in this book. You can learn the same approaches that Sarah learned in her class so you can explore the possibility of a life with a better resilience against stress. The journey will not always be easy, but I will do my best to encourage you to keep taking the next step.

First, however, is stress the problem you're struggling with?

Have you been thinking in any of the following ways?

- Constant worrying
- Predicting the worst
- Racing mind
- Negative thinking

Have you had any of the following feelings?

- Low mood
- Sense of inadequacy

- Anxiety
- Frustration
- Panic

Have you had any of the following physical symptoms?

- Headaches
- Stomach or bowel problems
- Sweating
- Feeling dizzy
- Breathlessness
- Sexual problems

Have you been acting in any of the following ways?

- Forgetful or clumsy
- Unsociable
- Eating more or less than usual
- Always busy
- Smoking or drinking more
- Exploding with anger

All of these are the symptoms of too much stress, a phenomenon that affects your thoughts, emotions, physical well-being, and behavior. However, there may be a medical reason for your symptoms, so some caution is required. Stress can creep up on you gradually and end up weighing heavily on you, to the point where every day feels like a struggle. You may intuitively know that there are two ways to relieve the burden of stress: eliminate the stressors in your life or reduce their effects on you. **This book can help you with both, by helping you adopt the new way of life Sarah learned, called** *mindful living.*

Mindfulness can help you reduce stress by developing a new level of awareness of:

- the **thoughts** that trigger the stress response
- the **emotions** (yours and others') that can bubble into conflict
- the **physical signs** that your body is in distress
- the **behaviors** that might be contributing to heightened stress as well as those that help you relax.

The stress response is complicated, and mindfulness is profoundly nuanced and powerful. Chapter 1 explains in more detail how mindfulness is ideally suited to help control the stress in your life. This book takes advantage of these benefits by presenting a self-help version of mindfulness-based stress reduction (MBSR), an 8-week mindfulness course originated in 1979 and usually done in a group setting with an MBSR teacher that has now been completed by hundreds of thousands of people. MBSR is the most well-researched mindfulness course in the world, so it makes sense to start there if stress is a problem for you.

The aim of the course is to teach a range of different mindfulness exercises and meditations to help reduce your stress in the long term. The course also offers a chance to explore mindful attitudes and values so you can meet future life challenges in a way that reduces rather than increases your stress. Finally, MBSR offers you a way of living so you can notice and take pleasure in the simple things in life that we all take for granted, and, in doing so, focus on what's going well in your life, not just what's going wrong, no matter how bad things seem.

When Dr. Jon Kabat-Zinn and colleagues at the University of Massachusetts Medical School designed MBSR, the goal was to make the benefits of traditional Buddhist mindfulness meditation accessible in a secular way to people suffering from chronic pain and other long-term health conditions. The program was designed to include not only meditation but also yoga, models about stress, group discussion, and ways of integrating mindfulness into daily life. All of these except the group discussion are offered in this book, and throughout, you'll read composite stories about and quotes representative of what I've heard from people who have reduced their stress levels using MBSR to replicate the group experience.

I discovered MBSR when I was researching the scientific basis of meditation. I attended an MBSR class in London and was impressed by the format and secular approach. I longed to share this course with others, and so I began my training in MBSR with Jon Kabat-Zinn and Saki Santorelli through the Center for Mindfulness at the University of Massachusetts Medical School. I then studied how to teach MBSR for several years at Bangor University's Centre for Mindfulness in the United Kingdom. I began teaching MBSR to people suffering from stress in my local area, both in small groups and one on one. Over several years, I taught many MBSR groups, mainly to members of the public who wanted to discover a different way of handling their stress. Then I published my first book on the subject. This led to invitations to give talks and workshops in mindfulness around the world—a real privilege. I now also run online mindfulness teacher training programs and various other online offerings. I also continue to deliver workshops when offered the opportunity.

How to Use This Book

This book is not a workbook but a practical manual. Eight chapters take you through the 8-week program with full instructions for what to do and when to do it. I encourage you to use a journal—whether a book to write in or your tablet, phone, or computer—to record your reflections about your experiences with the program and how it affects your stress levels. Having a written record gives you something to refer back to to refine your practice in the days and years to come. Your journal can also shift your mindful living in ways that will work even better for you than what you tried first. Finally, keeping a written record can remind you of all the good things in your life that mindfulness helps you recognize, along with the challenges.

I've also provided downloadable audio tracks for the meditation practices, available at *www.guilford.com/alidina-materials*. (If at any time you feel the need to practice the mindfulness meditations without guidance, there is a set of tracks, numbers 21–24, with only intermittent bells every 5 or 10 minutes to remind you to be mindful. Use these tracks whenever you prefer them to a guided mindfulness audio.)

After reading about exactly how mindfulness reduces stress in Chapter 1, Chapters 2 and 3 will help you look more closely at your own stress levels right now (including whether your stress is severe enough that it would be wise to get professional help) and lay out how to work through the program. But please don't take the word "work" too seriously. I've offered two routes through the course—a mini-version ⏱ and a full version ⏱—so that you can adapt the program to your own needs and desires and ensure that the program actually reduces your stress rather than adds to it. I've also included an illustrated chapter of mini and full mindful yoga exercises that I will refer to throughout the book. At the back of the book you'll find a lot of resources that will lead you to more information, more help, and allow you to read the full reports of the research studies discussed in the book if you like.

Life can be tremendously stressful, and there are many ways to cope with that pressure. I'm honored that you're considering "walking" with me to understand and develop greater mindful awareness. Thank you for your attention so far, and I sincerely hope that you find that the flexible course in this book eases your stress and enriches your life.

ONE

How Mindfulness Helps with Stress

There is a saying in Tibetan: "Tragedy should be utilized as a source of strength." No matter what sort of difficulties, how painful experience is, if we lose our hope, that's our real disaster.

—DALAI LAMA

AS SARAH began to practice mindfulness exercises, she became more aware of how wild her mind was. All kinds of thoughts, many unconnected to what she was attempting to focus on, entered and exited her mind. She also noticed how negative many of these thoughts were: "I'm useless" and "What's wrong with me?" and "I can't cope with this job and all the other stuff going on." These thoughts kept going around and around in her head. Through mindfulness, she learned to step back from the thoughts in her mind so that they gradually had less of an impact on her feelings of stress.

As her head began to feel a bit clearer, she felt more in control. She found herself less reactive when her son didn't do as he was told. She could see why he was acting out—he hadn't eaten for hours or was tired after school. She felt more compassion for him, and he responded more positively to her calmer tone of voice.

Sarah also felt less tired at work due to an improved ability to focus, and so managed to work more efficiently and leave the office earlier.

In the evenings, when she got home from work, she did a short mindfulness exercise. This helped her shift out of work mode and be more calm and relaxed at home. She learned not to feel so guilty when doing nothing; just sitting down and resting or playing with her son was okay, she realized. In fact, it was essential.

Everyone has a wild mind. We all overreact to the demands of our lives when stretched to our limits. Our world collapses in on itself and we lose empathy for others who are struggling just as we are when stress has us in its grip. It's not our fault—it seems to be the way nature made us. Fortunately, we need not lose hope that things can get better. Sarah's story illustrates that, although mindfulness begins slowly and it's not a quick, smooth ride to an instant stress-free life, if you practice, mindfulness can slowly and steadily soothe your mind and heart, positively nourishing all parts of your life. It's a bit like gentle rain soaking into a land of drought. The rain is mindfulness. The drought is the constant doing of modern living.

To understand how mindfulness can relieve stress, we need to take a closer look at what stress is.

What Exactly Is Stress?

Here's a definition:

> Stress is the feeling of being
> under too much pressure.

Pressure can be classified as external (in the world around you) or internal (your thoughts, emotions, and attitudes).

Examples of external pressures include:

- Having to complete work
- Having to do chores and take care of other tasks at home
- Taking care of yourself and those around you
- Having to travel to work or social events
- Managing your own illness or the illness of others
- E-mails, phone calls, and other communications
- Child rearing
- Needing to exercise
- Lacking money

Examples of internal pressures include:

- Negative, judgmental thoughts about yourself
- Negative, judgmental thoughts about others
- Negative thoughts or ideas about the world

- Low self-esteem or low self-compassion
- A tendency toward perfectionism
- Difficult emotions such as depression, anxiety, anger, guilt, or shame that linger for weeks
- Discomfort or pain in your body

You need some external pressure to motivate and excite you. If the pressure is too low for you, you'll feel bored or useless. If the pressure is too high for you, you'll experience high levels of stress. In some ways, your life is a balancing act of finding activities that offer the right level of pressure for *you*. Everyone's different and at any one time we all require different levels of pressure, whether it's internal or external, to live optimally.

> If the pressure is too high for you and lasts for long periods of time, it can cause chronic stress, and that's where the danger lies.

The pressures you experience may not be much higher than you can cope with. But over long periods of time, they can cause problems. For example, imagine I asked you to hold a glass of water out in front of you. If you had to hold the glass of water for a minute, you'd have no problem. You could easily smile at the same time. If you had to hold the glass for 10 minutes, the task becomes trickier, and you may not be smiling so much, but you could manage. But if I asked you to hold that glass of water all day and all night, I'd probably have to call an ambulance by the end of the day.

The glass of water represents the pressure you face. As you can see, the pressure in itself wasn't the issue; the issue was how long you were subjected to it. The duration of the pressure raised its level to the point where it caused stress. This shows how peaks of pressure now and then are not harmful, but long-term pressure can turn to stress.

Having the right level of pressure leads to a life of greater happiness. If you're reading this book, I assume that you're currently under too much pressure rather than too little and will offer you ways to help ease that pressure.

What Toll Does Stress Take on Us?

Stress, or more accurately the stress response, causes changes to take place in your brain and body. These changes can cause various kinds of harm when stress becomes chronic:

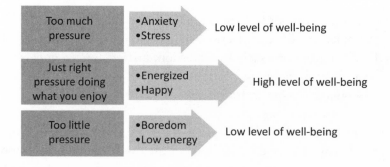

- Persistent stress can cause a range of **physical diseases**. Some estimate up to 75% of visits to the physician are stress related. Stress can cause high blood pressure, leading to heart problems including heart attacks. Stress can also cause migraines, back pain, and ulcers. Stress also weakens your immune system, making you susceptible to a range of diseases.
- Chronic stress affects your **mental well-being**. Stress can lead to clinical depression, anxiety, and burnout. Stress also reduces your ability to focus effectively.
- Stress affects your **family life**. When your stress levels are high, you're more likely to snap at your partner or children. If this happens too regularly, the quality of your relationship will diminish. Stress weakens your emotional intelligence, making it difficult to see things from other people's point of view.
- **Addiction** to illicit drugs, alcohol, or nicotine can be linked to chronic stress. You may be using these substances to help relieve the feeling of stress, although the relief is short lived and the addiction raises the overall level of stress.
- **Society as a whole** suffers from stress. The cost to each nation due to reduced efficiency or missing work because of stress runs into hundreds of billions of dollars. And that doesn't touch on the reduced levels of creativity and communication issues due to excessive stress levels.

How Can Mindfulness Reduce Stress?

Stress is a complex subject, and so the path to relieving it is not straightforward either, as Sarah discovered. However, for the sake of simplicity, here are some ways mindfulness helps you with stress.

- You become more **aware of your thoughts**. You can then step back from them and not take them so literally. That way, your stress response is not initiated in the first place.

- **You don't immediately react** to a situation. Instead, you have a moment to pause and then use your "wise mind" to come up with the best solution. Mindfulness helps you do this through the mindful exercises.
- **Mindfulness switches on your "being" mode** of mind, which is associated with relaxation. Your "doing" mode of mind is associated with action and the stress response.
- You are more **aware and sensitive to the needs of your body**. You may notice pains earlier and can then take appropriate action.
- You are **more aware of the emotions of others**. As your emotional intelligence rises, you are less likely to get into conflict.
- **Your level of care and compassion for yourself and others rises**. This compassionate mind soothes you and inhibits your stress response.
- Mindfulness practice **reduces activity in the part of your brain called the amygdala**. The amygdala is central to switching on your stress response, so effectively, your background level of stress is reduced.
- **You are better able to focus**. So you complete your work more efficiently, you have a greater sense of well-being, and this reduces the stress response. You are more likely to get into "the zone" or "flow," as it's termed in psychology by Mihaly Csikszentmihalyi.
- **You can switch your attitude to the stress**. Rather than just seeing the negative consequences of feeling stressed, mindfulness offers you the space to think differently about the stress itself. Observing how the increased pressure helps energize you has a positive effect on your body and mind.

Later in this chapter I describe in detail how mindfulness can benefit you physically, mentally, emotionally, and in your relationships. First, however, it's important to understand the difference between our typical mental state, mindlessness, and mindfulness.

> "The mindfulness course made me realize I'd been sleepwalking my whole life. Stress reduction was just one of the many benefits of mindfulness for me."

Mindlessness: The Usual Mode of Mind

Your normal state of mind during routine activities is probably a state of mindlessness. I don't mean to be accusatory or rude—it's just what the brain defaults to. In the mindless state, you are living a life of unconscious habits. You don't give full attention to every activity you do, but just go through the motions.

Your brain is designed to form habits. This process can help you complete tasks more efficiently. A habit is actually the process of the neurons in your brain connecting to each other due to regular firing down a particular pathway. You can think of each habit as a computer program. It takes place automatically and quickly and doesn't require any conscious awareness. The habits are formed through a process of repetition. Each time you repeat an activity, you're beginning to create that habitual program. Habits have several benefits:

- The activity can be done unconsciously so you use up less energy in your conscious awareness. You do not need to think "move left leg, move right leg" when walking. It just happens.
- You don't need to waste energy making choices. You wake up and brush your teeth—you don't need to decide to brush your teeth today.
- Habitual activities can be done much more quickly. Doing something new, like playing the piano, is far more difficult and slow at the beginning.
- You feel more relaxed. You're not trying hard to engage in the habit—it happens by itself. If you have a habit of eating an apple a day, you don't need to try hard to force yourself to eat the healthy fruit.
- You can be more effective in your activity. When you first try to juggle, it's difficult and you keep dropping the balls. Once it's an automatic action, you can hop on one leg and tell a joke at the same time.

However, there are several disadvantages of habits too:

- As habits are normally unconscious, you're not awake to the experience. If you're playing with your child habitually, you miss the special and precious moment of being together. The experience can't be savored if habitual.
- You lose choice. How can you make a choice if you're acting automatically and habitually? If you've always traveled from San Francisco to Chicago by plane, you book the ticket automatically. You don't consider a train journey or a road trip with friends.
- When your thoughts, emotions, and attitudes are both habitual and negative, you're much more likely to experience stress. Persistent unmindful, negative thinking turns on your stress response.

> Habitual negative thoughts about yourself, others,
> and the world are at the root of a lot of stress.
> Mindfulness helps you undo those unhelpful habits

and to rewire your brain to generate greater happiness
and less chronic stress.

PRACTICE: Two-Minute Mindfulness Exercise

Audio track 1: 2 minutes.

Try this exercise right now.

1. Set a timer for 2 minutes.
2. Begin by taking a deep, slow breath in and out.
3. Now pay attention to the **feeling** of your breathing. Just breathe naturally. Each time you notice your mind drift to other thoughts, gently bring your attention back to your breath.
4. After 2 minutes, you can stop.

Reflection

Give yourself a few moments to reflect on the following questions. If you feel like writing them down, you can enter your answers in your smartphone or tablet (if you have one). Once you start the 8-week program, you'll be encouraged to acquire a journal or start recording these reflections electronically in one place, so you can get a jump on the journaling now if you like.

1. What did you notice?
2. Were you able to focus your attention on your breathing?
3. Where else did your attention wander to?
4. How did you feel at the end of the exercise?
5. Was it easy or difficult?

Remember: Your mind will drift to other thoughts. This is normal. It doesn't mean you're doing anything wrong. In fact, if you noticed that your mind drifted, it means you're doing the exercise correctly.

Now repeat the experiment, but this time try sitting or standing up straight and close your eyes if they were open the first time. Then reconsider the questions above. Which of the two exercises was it easier to focus in?

Understanding Mindfulness

Mindfulness is the opposite of habitual, automatic living. Mindfulness teaches you to live more consciously. You still have your habits, because that is the nature of the brain, but you notice them more and gain greater choice in your life.

Here's my definition of mindfulness, which brings together the essence of the many different definitions that mindful teachers have shared:

> Mindfulness means intentionally paying attention
> to your present-moment experience
> with mindful attitudes such as acceptance, curiosity,
> self-compassion, and openness.

Let's break this definition down to make better sense of its meaning.

INTENTIONALLY

Mindfulness isn't usually an automatic process. You don't often find yourself being mindful. Mindfulness is a process that requires a decision; you need to choose to be mindful. And then you exert a certain kind of effort, at least initially. Once you begin to get into the flow of mindful awareness, your level of effort may decrease, but at least initially, there is a purposeful decision to pay attention.

Interestingly, you're paying attention to something almost all the time. The question is what you're paying attention to. While reading this book, your mind may be on the television on in the background. Or thinking about what's going to happen at work today. Or replaying what happened yesterday. This is passive attention. Passive attention is involuntary. Mindfulness is more than just paying attention passively to wherever your attention goes.

Mindfulness is an active rather than passive attention. An active, or purposeful, attention requires choice and a certain degree of effort. We get into intention in more detail later in this chapter.

PAYING ATTENTION

You can think of attention as a focused awareness. The word attention comes from the Latin *attendere*, meaning literally "to stretch toward." When you pay attention to a lecture, you're stretching your awareness toward the speaker's voice.

Attention is about taking notice—being aware of what's happening while it's happening. We use our senses to pay attention to external experiences: sights, sounds, smells, tastes, touch. You can pay attention to, for example, the sight of this book, the sound of a baby crying in the distance, the smell of oil from a deep fryer in a fast-food restaurant, the taste of your morning orange juice, and the sensation of the weight of your body on your chair, or tension in your shoulders. When you pay attention to these experiences purposefully, you're being mindful.

But you're not restricted to your outer senses in mindfulness. Consciously focusing on your internal experiences such as your thoughts and emotions without being swept away by them, as best you can, is mindfulness. You can pay attention to thoughts like "I can't be bothered to do this job" or "Why is that woman shouting?" or emotions like boredom, excitement, or frustration. To notice these internal experiences rather than just **unconsciously having** them, is mindfulness. That little sense of separation between you and your thoughts or emotions is key.

You may think, "So what? Okay, so I'm not 100% aware all the time. I daydream. I think about other stuff. What's wrong with that?" Well, here's a typical example of an experience I had last week. Imagine you were on this business trip: You wake up ready to get a flight back home from a business trip, from Chicago to London. You check the weather and discover the forecast is not good. Twelve inches of snow is predicted. The report says lots of flights will either be delayed or canceled. You think, "Oh no! My flight's gonna be canceled. I was really looking forward to getting back home and spending some time with the kids before going back to work. Why does this always happen to me? It's so annoying. Will I be able to get a hotel for an extra night? This airline always gives poor service when these things happen." You begin to feel tense and stressed.

Now consider an alternative scenario: You wake up, ready to get a flight back home from a business trip, from Chicago to London. You check the weather and discover the forecast is not good. Twelve inches of snow is predicted. The report says lots of flights will either be delayed or canceled. You think, "Oh no, my flight's gonna be canceled." Then you actually notice that you've had that particular thought. You recognize it as a prediction, not a fact. You then check your flight online and discover that it is actually flying and, with a bit of luck, you may take off on time. As you spend the morning in a coffee shop, you enjoy the beauty of the snow while sipping your cup of tea. You know that how much or little you worry will make no difference.

This is one example of mindfulness in action. By being aware of your thoughts, you're able to take action rather than allow your mind to run away with itself. The example shows the following key principle:

> Being unmindful actually causes you to suffer, often
> more than you think.

IN THE PRESENT MOMENT

Most young children have their attention drawn to the present moment. They are intensely curious. Children notice the sound of the plane, the bird in the tree, and the taste of the grapes. As they grow up, their memory is filled with experiences of the past, and they are able to project into the future. With this unique human ability, as we grow up, we tend to be less connected with the present moment.

Your mind seems to naturally replay past incidents and worry about the future. While reading this, you may find yourself thinking about that comment your friend made: Was she being rude?

Just as a swinging pendulum moves from left to right, spending little time in the middle, so your mind spends a lot of time in the past and future. In fact, research in 2010 by Killingsworth and Gilbert at Harvard University suggested the typical human brain spends about 50% of its time thinking about the past and future and only 50% in the here and now, the present moment.

Why is present-moment living important? The great leader Gandhi once said: "The future depends on what we do in the present moment." If your attention is excessively in the past and future, you can't perform effectively in the here and now, the present moment. But tomorrow never comes; there is only today. What you do today and how you focus now matters.

The following example illustrates this point. I was chatting with one of my clients, Katie, the other day. She told me that before she did a mindfulness course she was constantly worrying about her children and their future. Was she a good mother? Was she bringing up her children well, using the right parenting approach? She read websites and books, and they all seemed to give different advice. She felt lost and confused and very tired. After practicing mindfulness, Katie decided to let all those thoughts go and be present with her child. She gave her little boy her full attention, and her time with him felt so much more special. Her worrying receded, and she felt she was a much better mother when she was living in the present moment rather than worrying about what was right and wrong all the time.

Without conscious effort, your mind wanders to thoughts about the past or the future. And the thoughts about the past can easily end up being about negative interactions. You think about the argument you had with your brother for the tenth time or consider all the different reasons your new girlfriend isn't calling you.

Of course, there's nothing wrong with thinking. In fact, thinking is essential for survival as a human being in the modern age. The problem is the constant worrying that leads to unhappiness. Mindfulness helps to bring some balance back from relentless thinking, worrying, and planning.

MINDFUL ATTITUDES OF ACCEPTANCE, CURIOSITY, SELF-COMPASSION, AND OPENNESS

Mindfulness is more than just paying attention. It's also about paying attention with the right attitude. If your attention is infused with negativity, self-criticism, and judgment, it's not likely to be beneficial. You need to bring certain attitudes, what I call mindful attitudes, so that you build your attention on a positive foundation. All these attitudes don't have to be cultivated perfectly and don't need to be kept in your conscious awareness all the time. They are the flavoring in the soup of mindful awareness that you're cooking. Any one of them is more than satisfactory in a mindfulness exercise that you do. You'll learn a lot more about each of these attitudes as you read through this book.

Tales of Wisdom: The Anger-Eating Monster

Once upon a time, there was a king who lived in a beautiful palace. The king had to go away for a while, and while he was away, a monster approached the gates of the palace. The monster was so ugly and smelly, and his words so disgusting, that the guards froze in shock. He passed the guards and sat on the king's throne. The guards soon came to their senses, went in, and shouted at the monster, demanding that he get off the throne. With each foul word they used, the monster grew more smelly, ugly, and disgusting. The guards got even angrier—they began to brandish their swords and use violence to remove the monster. But the monster just grew bigger and bigger, eventually taking up the whole room. He grew more smelly, ugly, and disgusting than ever. He was smellier than the restrooms in the roughest bar on a drunken Saturday night.

Eventually the king returned. He was wise and kind and saw what was happening in the confrontation. He knew what to do. He smiled and said "Welcome to my palace!" to the monster. He then asked the monster if anyone had offered him a cup of coffee. The monster began to grow smaller as he sipped the drink. The king offered him some take-out pizza and fries. The guards immediately called for pizza. The monster continued to shrink with the king's kind gestures. The king then offered the monster a full body massage, and as the guards helped with the relaxing massage, the monster became tiny. With a final act of kindness to the monster, he just disappeared.

The source of your stress may be an anger-eating monster. Do you think your anger is making your anger-eating monster bigger? With some stressful circumstances, the more negative thoughts, words, or actions you have, the more difficult the situation becomes. Perhaps this story may help you open your heart to your challenge and see the value of a more friendly approach? Just being friendly toward yourself may be what's required.

The Physical Benefits of Mindfulness

Although mindfulness is often referred to as a form of mind training, the approach has many physical benefits. This is often because mindfulness reduces excessive stress, and stress is associated with many physical ailments.

Here are some of the key positive effects of practicing mindfulness exercises and meditations on a regular basis.

MORE RELAXED MUSCLES

When you become stressed, your muscles tighten up. There's a reason for this. Stress engages your body's fight-or-flight response. Your muscles are preparing to work hard to enable you to run away or fight. Mindfulness helps you notice the tension in your body as one sign that your stress levels are rising. With this awareness you can begin taking action to reduce the stress. In addition, the very awareness of the tension often reduces it.

I remember working with a woman who suffered from what she called chronic tension. Her whole body was so tense that moving was painful and sometimes impossible. Traditional relaxation exercises didn't seem to help her. But by learning mindfulness she learned to become aware of that physical tension without trying to change it. She learned to be a little less judgmental and a little more accepting of the sensations. This led to an easing and reduction in that tension and a reduction in pain.

A HEALTHIER HEART

When you're stressed, your heart beats faster and your blood pressure rises to prepare you to run or fight. Your body reacts as if you're under attack. Heart disease is the number-one cause of death in Americans each year, and anxiety is one of the contributing factors. Initial indications showed that for a group suffering from heart disease, mindfulness helped. The group had a reduction in anxiety, improved ability to manage emotions, and a better style of coping with stress and took more effective control of their health.

AN IMPROVED RELATIONSHIP WITH FOOD

Do you have trouble digesting your food? Another problem with the stress response is your digestive system stops working effectively. Your body is reacting as if it's about to be eaten by a tiger. If you're going to end up as someone else's lunch, there's no point wasting your energy digesting your own breakfast. Lowering stress through efforts like mindfulness can ease digestive distress. Applying mindfulness specifically to eating also prepares your body to digest: being more conscious as you eat, you taste your food and avoid multitasking, and your brain sends the appropriate messages to your digestive system to begin its work. This is mindful eating. Studies have shown mindful eating can reduce bingeing and overeating, can help you lose weight, can reduce chronic conditions like anorexia and bulimia, and help with the symptoms of Type 2 diabetes.

A LONGER LIFE—THROUGH PROTECTION OF YOUR DNA

This is an incredible finding. Just as the ends of shoelaces have a tip to protect them from fraying, so the chromosomes in your cells have a cap on them to stop them from fraying. These protective caps are called telomeres. Before it was thought that the wearing out of these caps was inevitable, resulted in cells dying, eventually leading to death of the cell due to "old age." But in 2009, Dr. Elizabeth Blackburn won the Nobel Prize for discovering that a substance in the body called telomerase protects the telomeres. More telomerase would mean a longer life. And here comes the good news: mindfulness increases the amount of telomerase. This helps to effectively reduce or perhaps reverse the aging of your cells. So be mindful and look young and vibrant!

BETTER IMMUNE FUNCTION

One other key function that gets almost shut down when you're stressed is your immune system. Your immune system is a long-term protective system but gets overridden by the stress response, which is your short-term survival mechanism. If you're chronically stressed, you're much more likely to get sick. Research by Professor Richard Davidson from the University of Wisconsin and colleagues found that, following an 8-week mindfulness course, participants produced more antibodies to fight flu compared with those who hadn't gone through the mindfulness course. Other research has shown mindful practitioners miss fewer days of work due to respiratory infections and have milder symptoms for a shorter time.

A 2009 study of 48 people who tested HIV positive showed mindfulness may be very beneficial. The group that did an 8-week meditation course had no reduction in the number of white blood cells—a key part of the immune system. However, the nonmeditating group's level of white blood cells went down.

PAIN RELIEF—MORE THAN MORPHINE

A small study published in *Journal of Neuroscience* in 2011 found mindfulness reduced pain intensity by 40%. That's even more effective than morphine! The research found this pain relief seemed to be due to a different way your brain works after becoming more mindful. The researchers trained the participants in mindfulness for 1 hour and then asked them to practice mindfulness while they heated a small part of their skin to 120°F for 5 minutes—a painful experience for most people! Several other studies have found that mindfulness helped people manage not only acute pain but also chronic pain.

IMPROVED SLEEP

I find this is one of the first benefits that people mention when they begin practicing mindfulness, and there's research to back up their claims. Research from the University of Utah found mindfulness helped people regulate their emotions during the day and experience "lower activation" at bedtime, which may boost the quality of sleep.

Considering that you spend about a third of your life asleep, practicing mindfulness just to sleep better makes sense, but it also can help reduce stress. Mindfulness reduces your stress and thereby improves your sleep. The improvement in sleep in turn makes you feel even less stressed. The mindfulness begins a positive feedback loop.

Benefits for Your Brain and Mind

These are the benefits of mindfulness that most people are familiar with, particularly the way mindfulness improves focus and helps to calm your mind. But there's more to mindfulness than that! Here's what the research shows.

A CLEARER MIND

Several studies have shown that mindfulness practice reduces rumination or worrying. Research in 2009 published in the *Journal of Science and Healing* found participants of an 8-week MBSR course had greater levels of well-being and reduced rumination. In my experience, one of the beneficial side effects is creativity. When I practice mindfulness, I often end up having ideas that help in my daily work or home life. The title for this very book came up for me in a meditation while attending a retreat.

A CALMER MIND

Many studies have proven the stress reduction effects of mindfulness. That's obviously what this book is all about. Exactly why mindfulness reduces stress is actually unknown. One fascinating study, published in 2010 in the journal *Emotion*, explored the subject through the use of film. Two groups were asked to watch a sad movie. One group had completed an MBSR course, and the other had not. Brain scans reveal that the meditators had less brain activity compared to the nonmeditators, and the brain activity was distinctly different compared to the brain activity before doing the mindfulness training. This seems to suggest that mindfulness enables emotions to be processed differently in the brain and may be one way stress is reduced through mindfulness practice.

BETTER MEMORY

In particular, mindfulness boosts a type of memory that we all have called *working memory*. Think of your working memory as being like a little whiteboard. You use the whiteboard to make notes about what people are saying to you and what you need to do at the moment. A weak working memory is like having a very small whiteboard. You easily forget what you're doing and get distracted by other things. A larger whiteboard means you can remember what you're doing and remain less distracted by other people or thoughts. Stress has been shown to reduce working memory capacity, and mindfulness has been shown to increase working memory capacity. So mindfulness makes your little whiteboard a bit bigger. Improved working memory is associated with improved learning ability, focus, and skill in regulating emotions.

IMPROVED FOCUS

As you may have guessed, mindfulness improves your ability to focus. In fact, it improves focus a lot. Research in 2009 at Liverpool John Moores University found mindfulness meditators perform significantly better than nonmeditators in all measures of attention. When you focus better, you are more likely to get into a "flow" state of mind, an absorbed mental mode associated with high levels of well-being—the opposite of excessive stress. Improved focus also leads to a greater sense of achievement and greater efficiency, so more time for friends and family. You feel more in control rather than out of control.

Emotional Benefits

HAPPINESS!

Call it happiness, well-being, or flow—mindfulness helps to raise it. The sense that you are happy is linked to so many other benefits, including improved relationships, longer life, and better performance and outcomes at work. Plus, being happy feels good. The effect of mindfulness on happiness was found in research published in the *Journal of Behavioral Medicine* in 2008. The scientists found higher levels of well-being for those who participated in the MBSR course. Those who did more meditation and yoga practice at home had higher levels of mindfulness and well-being. The previously mentioned research by Killingsworth and Gilbert also found that people whose minds wandered less were happier.

PROTECTION AGAINST DEPRESSION

One of the problems with chronic stress is the emergence of depression. The link between stress and depression is complex, but there's certainly a link. Chronic stress changes the hormones in your bloodstream, making depression more likely. And when you're under too much pressure, you're less likely to socialize, eat healthily, or exercise—you can end up not looking after yourself. According to the World Health Organization, more than 350 million people suffer from depression and it's the leading cause of disability worldwide. Here in the United Kingdom, mindfulness is used to treat recurring clinical depression by the National Health Service (NHS). A group course in mindfulness called mindfulness-based cognitive therapy, which is similar in many ways to the course in this book, has been found to be 50% more effective than the usual treatments. Mindfulness helps you stop fighting the feeling of sadness. Instead you learn to accept the feeling, notice the associated thoughts and physical sensations, with compassion toward yourself. This shift helps to prevent sadness from being prolonged and intensified and becoming depression.

REDUCTION IN LONELINESS

One of the key factors that raises stress in older adults is loneliness. Humans are social beings, and without social contact feelings of loneliness can become overwhelming. Programs designed to increase social contact in older adults have so far been unsuccessful. Recent research at Carnegie Mellon University has found mindfulness meditation helped to reduce loneliness. Interestingly, they also found a reduction in the expression of a gene associated with inflammation. So mindfulness was affecting their genes. Inflammation is associated with cancer, cardiovascular diseases, and neurodegenerative diseases, so a reduction in this gene expression is a very promising finding too.

LESS ANXIETY

Anxiety is the feeling of fear, tension, or worry often caused by a stressful event. Stress isn't a diagnosable mental disorder, but anxiety can be. An anxiety disorder develops when your fight-or-flight system is switched on most of the time and you feel fear to an extent that it affects your everyday ability to function. In the past, treatment involved trying to change thoughts. But with mindfulness, the idea is to change your *relationship* to thoughts and move from avoiding feelings to approaching them. In 2012, researchers at the University of Bergen in Norway looked at 19 different studies and found mindfulness-based approaches to offer robust and substantial reductions in anxiety.

LOWER ANGER LEVELS

Anger arises when things are not going the way you want them to. Sometimes that anger is unnecessary and unhelpful. Frequent anger can be very destructive to your work and home life, increasing your stress. When you're feeling stressed, you're much more likely to get angry too. It's been found that anger is fueled by "hot thoughts"—negative, aggressive thinking patterns. Mindfulness helps you notice and reduce unhelpful thinking patterns and so can reduce your feelings of anger when appropriate. This research was published in the journal *Aggressive Behavior* back in 2010.

Relationship Benefits

Relationships matter—a lot. Human relationships have been shown in study after study to be the number-one factor that increases happiness. People with lots of good-quality relationships, and that includes friends or family members, are likely to have a higher resilience toward stress. This is because when difficulties arise in their lives, they have someone to talk to.

Mindfulness gives you a chance to increase the quality of your relationships with your friends, family, and colleagues via the mechanisms described below. And by increasing the quality of those relationships, you increase your resilience to stress—and that of the other people in your life, because you give them someone to talk to as well!

A PRESENT-MOMENT AWARENESS

When others are talking to you, how present are you? You may be with them physically, but are you with them mentally and emotionally?

I remember a manager I once had who was rarely focused when I spoke to him. At work parties, he would be looking over my shoulder. In meetings, he wouldn't acknowledge what I said to him. And he seemed to have his favorites on the team and others whom he didn't seem to care much about. This made him rather unpopular in the office, and his team felt unmotivated and frustrated as a result.

Being more present means you listen more effectively and the other person feels heard. And being heard is what others really want. You strengthen the relationship each time you are present.

MAKING CONSCIOUS CHOICES IN THE HEAT OF THE MOMENT

"Autopilot is the big enemy of relationships," according to Marsha Lucas, author of *Rewire Your Brain for Love.* The way we behave in relationships often flows from the way our brain was wired in early childhood. If you allow yourself to behave automatically in your relationships, you're likely to repeat unhelpful patterns. Mindfulness rewires your brain—including parts of the brain responsible for emotional regulation and self-awareness. Through this rewiring, you're less likely to react in knee-jerk fashion when faced with a difficult emotion. By being mindful, you can manage your emotions in the heat of the moment, as your brain would be better wired to manage that. Imagine the amount of stress that can be reduced by being less reactive and to make a more controlled choice of words and action when upset by a partner, family member, or colleague.

KINDNESS

Bringing a sense of kindness, compassion, or friendliness to your dealings with others is bound to increase the quality of your relationship. This will make you and the other person feel happier and more relaxed, reducing your levels of stress too. However, you need to balance kindness toward others with kindness toward yourself.

Last week a friend and colleague asked me to give a lecture on using mindfulness to overcome depression. Mindfulness is a wonderful, drug-free way of managing depression, and I was delighted to share my passion for this boon. However, I already had several other deadlines to meet that week. I had to be kind to myself on this occasion and say no to my friend. It wasn't easy. I don't like to say no to opportunities to speak about mindfulness, but if I didn't say no, I'd be denying myself rest. And by resting I was giving myself time to reduce my own stress, thereby preparing to offer a better service to others in the future.

Reflection

Consider your own life. Think about the last three things you said yes to. Were you being kind to yourself or to others? Then think about the last three things you said no to. Were you being kind to yourself or others? Record your answers in a print or electronic journal if you like.

Ideally, you want to have a balance. If you're always giving and too kind to others to the detriment of your own stress levels, think about saying no more often. And if you always look out for yourself and rarely care for others, consider reaching out and performing an act of kindness for someone else.

BEING NONJUDGMENTAL

Letting go of judgment is a great way to improve your relationships and reduce your stress. The key, if you do need to judge, is to judge the *action* and not the person. I like to think of the essence of all humans as pure and complete— just as they were as babies. But due to misunderstandings, past experiences, brain chemicals, or other influences, the other person doesn't always behave reasonably or compassionately.

Here's an example of how I've tried to apply this. I had a friendship for a couple of years that didn't end well. Mike and I used to go to the movies or theater together, meet up every week, share ideas, and generally support each other. Mike and I were good friends. Then one day, out of the blue, he accused me of not being a friend. He claimed I had ignored him at a party. Described how I had offered a new project to another friend before I offered it to him. He said he wanted to get things out in the open rather than hold them in. This was all out of the blue. A bit shocked, I accepted the criticisms and apologized. I had no idea he was having these feelings. Yet I still never heard from him again. No more e-mails, phone calls, or texts. He didn't reply to anything. At first I felt sad and confused. Then I felt frustrated that he would do this to me. Eventually, however, I accepted the situation. The way I did this was by letting go of my judgment of him and also applying this personal principle of mine:

> People are always doing the best they can, with the level
> of understanding and motivation they have,
> at any given moment.

There was no point in my judging Mike as wrong or bad. He did what he did because of what he thought of me. He didn't want to discuss it further. By letting go of my judgment of him, I could relax and release the stress I had when I thought of him. I forgive him, because *he did what he thought was right*. That's understandable. That doesn't mean what he did was right or fair or even wise—but he did what he did for a reason. I can now feel grateful that he gave me the opportunity to practice forgiveness and wish him a more fulfilling experience with his other friendships.

Reflection

Is there someone in your life whom you feel you should stop judging? Is there someone causing you stress just as you think about him or her? Would it be helpful if you forgave the person but not the action? Could you consider appreciating the chance they've given you to practice the act of forgiveness?

Write your thoughts in your smartphone, tablet, or journal if you like. This is not easy and you may disagree with this approach to offenses you've suffered. But it's certainly worth reflecting on.

Mindfulness Is Bigger Than Meditation

There are only two ways to become more mindful:

1. Mindfulness meditation
2. Everyday mindfulness

Mindfulness meditation, a particular type of meditation, is where you make time to make your brain more mindful. Mindfulness meditation can be done for less than 5 minutes all the way up to about 45 minutes. The meditation involves practicing a particular technique, such as focusing on your breath, body, or sounds.

Mindfulness meditation creates positive changes in your brain. It actually rewires your brain so that you're more happy, focused, clear-headed, and open—in other words, more mindful! Meditation is the most powerful way to enhance your brain's ability to be mindful.

Yoga, tai chi, or other mind–body disciplines that are done with a full mindful awareness can also be classified as a mindfulness meditation.

> "I'm not the kind of person that likes to sit down and meditate. The fact that mindfulness can be practiced while I'm walking, cooking, or gardening makes it so portable and accessible for me."

Everyday mindfulness involves *living* in a mindful way. Each time you do an activity, if you *intentionally* give the process your full attention with mindful attitudes like curiosity and openness (this can also be called detachment or stepping back), you also enhance your brain's mindfulness.

Everyday mindfulness can be practiced at any time in your daily life. You can do mindful eating, mindful walking, and even simply mindful breathing while you're waiting in line somewhere. These types of everyday mindfulness are described in full throughout the 8-week program.

This is why mindfulness is bigger than meditation. Meditation can be practiced only at particular times in the day, when you make time to meditate. But you have the choice to be mindful at any moment in the day by giving full attention to whatever you're engaged in. Ready to discover what's so special about the 8-week mindfulness course in this book?

TWO

Discovering Mindfulness-Based Stress Reduction

Feelings come and go like clouds in a windy sky.
Conscious breathing is my anchor.
—THICH NHAT HẠNH

OMAR WAS lying in bed. He was in the hospital following a car accident. The nurse was doing a regular checkup and was watching his heart rate and blood pressure. Suddenly the nurse looked concerned. Her eyes locked onto the green computer screen connected to Omar by a spaghetti junction of wires. She looked back at Omar's face. He didn't seem pale; his eyes were closed, and he seemed like he was almost smiling. The nurse grew perplexed and decided to wake him up. She shook Omar's arm, and he calmly opened his eyes. "Your blood pressure just dropped a lot," she said. "I'm a bit worried. That doesn't normally happen so quickly. How are you feeling?" Omar smiled and said, "I'm listening to a mindfulness meditation from my old MBSR class" as he removed his earphones. "Your what class?" asked the nurse, smiling but confused. "It's a meditation course I did years ago. I still listen to the audio to help reduce my stress. That's probably why my blood pressure dropped!"

Although Omar had done the MBSR course years ago, he regularly practiced mindfulness. Over time, he became more skilled at being mindful and used the guided audio whenever he felt his stress levels rising. The MBSR program teaches you to identify moments in life when your stress levels are rising and offers simple exercises to help reduce that stress.

That's MBSR in a nutshell: learning through mindfulness to catch mounting stress and lower it before it takes hold. In this chapter I'll tell you a little about the history of the program and how it's structured.

Understanding MBSR

If you read Chapter 1, you know a bit about what mindfulness is and what the benefits of regular practice are, but it might be helpful to know how MBSR arose and how the group model on which this self-help book is based works. MBSR was designed to be taught as an 8-week course so that participants had the chance to try out the mindfulness exercises during the week. At the end of each session, the group would be given mindfulness experiments to try out. Then they could return for the next week's session and discuss what worked for them and what didn't seem to work. The same format is used today, and the course in this book takes 8 weeks too.

All MBSR teachers follow a standardized curriculum but teach the sessions in their own way. Some MBSR teachers may be a little more didactic; others prefer to open up for questions. Some MBSR teachers include lots of mindful yoga practice in their class; others may use other forms of mindful movement.

Regardless of these variations, all trained MBSR teachers are asked to include four fundamental mindfulness meditation practices. They are the body scan meditation, the expanding awareness meditation (sometimes just called *sitting meditation*), a mini-meditation (about 3 minutes), and mindful movement meditations (mindful walking, mindful yoga, or simply mindful stretching).

Each session of the MBSR course starts with a guided mindfulness meditation that lasts about 30 minutes. This is followed by a chance for participants to discuss and explore their experience, called "inquiry." Following the inquiry, the particular theme of the session is explained. Themes include topics like "living on automatic pilot," "dealing with difficulties," and "discovering acceptance." The emphasis is on learning through experience rather than just giving participants information to discuss intellectually.

MBSR was originally offered to people with a range of physical and psychological health conditions. The program has now been adapted for different contexts, such as the workplace or schools, and for different health conditions such as eating disorders or cancer. At its core, however, the MBSR course has changed very little from the time it was initially developed a few decades ago. The main change is probably the addition of the 3-minute mini-meditation, which many people find useful.

Although MBSR was initially designed for those suffering from a health condition, it is now offered to anyone who is suffering from stress and wants to learn mindfulness. With the current way the world seems to work, that means pretty much everyone! Even if you don't suffer from stress, MBSR can help protect you from future stressors too. Although the kind of stressors faced by people in the 1970s and '80s may be different from those faced by you and me today, the mindfulness exercises and meditations remain the same. In fact, the mindfulness meditations shared in MBSR are thousands of years old. Learning MBSR from this book is a different experience from being in a class. You can't discuss your ideas with a teacher or with other members of the group, nor can you easily be encouraged by classmates. However, with this book you can work at your own pace, you don't need to travel to learn the program, and if you feel too shy to learn mindfulness in a group setting, this book can be a great approach. (This book can be used not just as a standalone course, however, but also in conjunction with a teacher, therapist, or coach.)

In writing this book, I've done my best to capture the spirit of an MBSR class. I've included all the core mindfulness meditations and exercises that you'd encounter in a real class, and I've included a Q-and-A section to answer the typical questions that arise. I've also made one fundamental addition to the MBSR program.

Two Different Routes through This Book

This book contains two versions of the mindfulness exercises in MBSR. The first version, what I call "**mini**," consists of short mindfulness exercises I've developed for busy people who want the flavor of mindfulness in their life but don't have too much time. Doing this version of the program is like a mini-MBSR. The other version, labeled "**full**," has the deep mindfulness practices for those who have the time to do them. The full program is the typical MBSR program. You can pick and choose what sort of mindfulness exercise you want to do as you go through the book or decide to take one route or the other throughout.

Besides basing your choice on the time you have available, your lifestyle, and what you hope to get from the approach—and it's important to consider these factors; after all, you're trying to reduce stress, not add to it—you can select the mini or full course depending on your level of stress. If your ongoing stress level is generally mild yet persistent, the mini-course may be for you. If it's more serious, I recommend the full course. (Again, however, you can use exercises from both courses as desired and your other obligations allow.)

DEALING WITH LOW–LEVEL, PERSISTENT STRESS: WATCH FOR THE MINI SYMBOL

This is for the majority of people in our modern society. If you have a demanding job, or have a family to care for, you're likely to have very little spare time for yourself. With this kind of busy lifestyle, you're probably looking for mindfulness to help take the edge off the relentless stress that you're facing. Here's what I'd recommend:

- Work through the 8-week course by reading the material and practice the shorter meditations for the home practice.
- Focus on living in a mindful way. See Chapter 6, which gives examples of mindful walking. You could also practice mindful driving, mindful cleaning, or mindful working. This is the everyday mindfulness I mentioned earlier and takes up no extra time, so it may be ideal for you. See more in Chapter 6.
- Consider using alarms on your phone, apps, or setting an appointment with yourself to be mindful. For you, the main challenge will be to remember to practice mindfulness and finding and making the necessary time and finding the motivation to practice, however short that may be.

DEALING WITH CHRONIC, HIGH LEVELS OF STRESS: WATCH FOR THE FULL SYMBOL

You may be suffering from high levels of stress. Perhaps you even have clinical anxiety or depression. You may currently be on medication or have taken medication in the past to manage your health. Or maybe you have been diagnosed with an illness or a medical condition like high blood pressure and want to use mindfulness to deal with the stress associated with the disease. Whatever the reason, for you stress is significantly affecting your ability to engage in your daily activities or has become an almost life-threatening situation, and you are willing to make the time to fully reduce your stress using mindfulness.

Here's what I recommend, with permission from your health professional:

- Complete the full 8-week mindfulness course outlined in this book. Do the daily 30-minute meditations and other recommended exercises.
- Practice everyday mindfulness. Integrate mindfulness into all you do at work, at home, and while traveling. This may also include avoiding all forms of multitasking and slowing down your actions so they are more mindful. This will deepen your mindful awareness. You will probably find you'll get more done because the quality of your work will be more focused and attentive.
- Consider finding a mindfulness group or doing an online mindfulness course (I offer one at *www.livemindfulonline.com*) to supplement your

learning and be part of an online community if you can't find one in your area.

Not sure how severe your stress is? Here's a self-assessment you can start with:

Assessing Your Stress Level

You can use the questionnaire below to get a rough idea of your current level of stress and guide you in how to use this book. If you want a more detailed assessment, for which we didn't have space in this book, visit *www.guilford. com/alidina-materials.*

Answer the questions below with 0 = never, 1 = sometimes, or 2 = often.

1. In the last month, how often have you been upset because of something that happened unexpectedly?

    Never/Rarely (0)   Sometimes (1)   Often (2)

2. In the last month, how often have you felt out of control?

    Never/Rarely (0)   Sometimes (1)   Often (2)

3. In the last month, how often have you felt stressed?

    Never/Rarely (0)   Sometimes (1)   Often (2)

4. In the last month, how often have you felt unable to cope with what you had to do?

    Never/Rarely (0)   Sometimes (1)   Often (2)

5. In the last month, how often have you felt angry because things were happening that were out of your control?

    Never/Rarely (0)   Sometimes (1)   Often (2)

Now add up your scores and record the total.

0–3 = You seem to have low levels of stress at the moment. Mindfulness could be used to build your resilience to protect your from future stress. The mini version of the course in this book should be sufficient, although there is no reason you can't do the full version if you find yourself benefiting greatly from learning mindfulness.

4–6 = Your level of stress is moderately high. Mindfulness is likely to help you manage your feeling of stress and perhaps reduce the chance of ill health. At this level you probably should let other factors dictate which practices you do—mini or full. You can probably benefit from either program or a mix of the two.

7–10 = Your stress level appears to be high. Mindfulness could help you manage your stress. **If you feel your stress has been at a very high level for some time, I'd recommend you visit a physician** or take action to reduce the source of your stress as soon as possible, if you can. Your physician could help you determine whether your symptoms are due to stress or some other condition and offer you the best treatment. Also consider the online stress questionnaires for a more accurate assessment. Consider doing the full MBSR program described in this book.

Reflection

What are the main symptoms you've been suffering in the last couple of weeks? Would it be helpful for you to talk to a physician or other health professional to clarify the best next step for you? Write your thoughts down in a paper or electronic journal if you like.

Complete the test again after completing the mindfulness program in this book and see if your stress has gone down. If not, do consider continuing to practice mindfulness—the process takes time but can be long lasting if you take the time to do the practices.

Tales of Wisdom: "What Are You?"

When the Buddha achieved the state of enlightenment, people were amazed at his presence. There was a radiance about him that seemed so mysterious and beautiful. "Are you God?" someone asked. "No," he replied. "Are you a saint?" asked another. "No," came the response, in a serene voice. "Then what are you?" they asked, deeply curious. He answered: "I'm awake."

The word *Buddha* actually means "awake."

When Should You Start?

Now that you have an idea of how high your stress level is, you know whether you should see your physician before starting this course and what path you might want to take through the practices. But knowing how much stress you are feeling can also help you figure out exactly when to start the course to get the most out of it. You may think mindfulness is the best thing to learn if you're really stressed out or in the middle of moving or dealing with a very recent breakup. Well, perhaps, not actually. It's a question of timing.

Learning mindfulness can be a challenging practice for three reasons:

1. Mindfulness is about learning a skill, and any skill involves a certain amount of time, effort, and challenge. Think about the last time you learned a new skill—painting, driving, or parenting. I'm sure it wasn't a quick acquisition. The mini-exercises may make it easier for you to learn, but they still take some time.
2. Mindfulness requires a daily discipline that can be difficult for people to follow. Think back to the last time you had to study for a test or exam—it's not always easy to sit down and actually do the work.
3. Mindfulness is about turning your attention inward, and although doing so is healthy, it can initially be unsettling if you're currently going through a lot of difficulties and aren't ready to deal with the emotions that may come up at first.

I'm obviously not trying to put you off doing mindfulness. I'd love everyone to learn mindfulness right away! But that's just not realistic. Being prepared for the challenges and picking the right time to learn is key to your success with mindfulness.

So when is a good time to go through a mindfulness course? Well, consider the following points to help you decide whether right now is the best time for you:

• **When you are not going through a major life change.** You need your life to be relatively stable before you start to learn mindfulness. If you are in the process of moving, changing jobs, or ending a relationship, this is probably not a great time to learn mindfulness. You're probably better off focusing your attention on sorting things out practically, so that when things are a little more settled, you have the time available to do the daily practices.

• **When you are in a relatively good state of mind.** Because mindfulness is a challenging practice, it's not recommended if you are in the midst of an episode of depression or high anxiety. If you wait for the episode to pass, you are more likely to be able to stick to the discipline of daily mindfulness and to finish the course. If you're not in a great place mentally, you may not finish the course and may classify your experience with mindfulness as another failure. Increase your chances of success by taking the course when you feel strong enough to do so. Of course, if your therapist or other health professional recommends a mindfulness course and will support you through it, using the right mindful exercises may be just what you need.

> "I really enjoyed doing the mini MBSR course in this book. The short meditations helped me to nip stress in the bud before it got out of control."

• **When you're fed up with the stress you're experiencing and ready to make a change.** You are, of course, welcome to simply read this book out of curiosity, without doing any of the practical exercises. If you're eager to reduce your stress, you'll need to do the recommended mindfulness exercises and meditations. If that sounds daunting, try the mini-exercises, which can help you dip your toe in to see if it's your sort of thing.

(TIP) If you really want to just read the book before doing any practices, that's fine. Do whatever you feel is right for you—my recommendations are just suggestions. You know what works best for you!

(TIP) If you think you're ready to try this course but not really feeling it fully, maybe all you need is a bit of a motivation boost. In that case you might opt for an in-person mindfulness course (see the Resources at the back of the book to find one near you), where you'll get encouragement and support from the other group members, or find a coach or mindfulness buddy. More on mindfulness buddies is on pages 43–44.

What Can You Expect?

Following is an outline of the MBSR course in this book. This will give you a little idea of the journey you can take as you go through the program.

WEEK 1: THERE'S MORE RIGHT WITH YOU THAN WRONG WITH YOU

In this session, you begin by discovering no matter how challenging your life circumstances are at the moment, there's more right than wrong with you. The session teaches you what mindfulness is, and you learn to practice the mindful body scan meditation. You also learn about automatic pilot—your mind's tendency to be unmindful and habitual for much of the day—and ways to turn it off (or at least tone it down).

WEEK 2: FROM AUTOMATIC REACTING TO CREATIVE RESPONDING

You explore the role of personal responsibility and interpretation in stress in this session. In addition to practicing the body scan again, you learn the mindful pause—a mini-meditation. You discover the link between thoughts and emotions and find some new ways of dealing with stressful thoughts.

WEEK 3: THE JOY AND VALUE OF LIVING IN THE PRESENT

In this session, you discover the true value of living in the present moment. You try the expanding awareness meditation, the body scan, and mindful movement practices to bring you into the here and now. You also discover how to enjoy mindful walking. Why your brain gets lost in stories, and how to come back to the present moment without judging yourself when this happens, is also covered.

WEEK 4: UNDERSTANDING AND MANAGING STRESS

Now you discover the physiology of stress. You find out how mindfulness helps you deal with stress and explore how to maintain peace in the face of unpleasant experiences. You continue to learn more mindful movement practices.

WEEK 5: TAKING A STAND—RESPONDING TO STRESS

Here you discover four key ways of dealing with stressors. You explore what it means to honor emotions rather than fight them. The session continues to teach ideas to help deepen your mindfulness meditation experience.

WEEK 6: MINDFUL COMMUNICATION

You explore mindfulness and its role in communication—different ways to apply mindfulness to listen deeply and speak effectively. You also discover the role of emotions and stress in communication and how to manage them using mindful attitudes and practices.

BETWEEN WEEKS 6 AND 7: A DAY OF MINDFULNESS

You find out the reasons for a day of mindfulness practice and explore the best ways to prepare for the day. You'll have the opportunity to decide what to do on your day of mindfulness, practicing the different mindfulness meditations you've learned. You'll also find out how to overcome common challenges that arise, such as dealing with emotions when practicing over an extended period of time.

WEEK 7: TAKING CARE OF YOURSELF

This session teaches you the importance of taking care of yourself when managing high levels of stress and how to use mindfulness to achieve this. You'll discover how to adjust your lifestyle to reduce stress, identifying the nourishing and depleting activities that can affect your stress levels, developing a mindful stress management action plan for dealing with stress, and discovering the mindful action step—a process of catching and overcoming stress before it spirals out of control.

WEEK 8: THE REST OF YOUR LIFE

The final session is an opportunity for reflection. You reflect on what you discovered in this course and how to continue practicing mindfulness. You uncover how to set your vision for a more mindful life with clear intentions for both the short and long term.

(TIP) If reading this has made you feel overwhelmed, please don't worry. Just take the course one day at a time and one practice at a time. The whole point is to be kind and gentle with yourself rather than feeling as if you're facing lots of things to "do."

INSIDE A SESSION

Here's what to expect in a typical session in this book:

1. Some mindfulness meditation practices to do
2. An explanation of the key themes of the session
3. Opportunities to reflect on your mindfulness meditation practice and the theme and to write about it in a journal (paper or electronic)
4. Some mindfulness home experiments to try out that week

Many of the practices that you'll be doing also give you the chance to do things a bit differently if you like.

VARIATION. These sections offer a different way of practicing the mindfulness exercise or meditation. You could experiment with these variations if you feel like trying something different.

GOING DEEPER. These sections give tips for more experienced mindfulness practitioners to do the meditations at a deeper level. You could use these tips if you choose to repeat this course on a second reading, for example, if you've already had some experience with mindfulness before applying it in MBSR.

How to Use This Book

I'd recommend you use this book in the following way:

1. Decide when you're ready to start your 8-week MBSR course, and when you're ready, read the next chapter to learn how to get the most out of the program.
2. As you read each week's chapter you'll be offered certain mindfulness practices. Do them before reading on for maximum benefit. It will probably take you 1–2 hours a week to read each chapter and do the exercises contained within the chapter.
3. You'll also be given certain reflective exercises to complete. Write down your answers in a journal or wherever you prefer.
4. In the week that follows, practice the mindfulness "home experiments" listed in the chart at the end of the chapter on a daily basis. This can range from 10 minutes to 30 minutes a day depending on what you prefer and your current stress levels and available time.
5. After a week of doing the home experiments, you're ready to move on to the next chapter.
6. If you didn't manage to do at least half of the daily practices for whatever reason, repeat that week before moving on to the next chapter.

TIP While I think you'll get the most out of each week's chapter if you stop and try the meditations while you're reading, feel free to read the whole chapter first and then go back and do the exercises. Whatever works best for you *is* best for you. You will definitely be better prepared to do the week's home experiments if you've already tried the practices during or right after reading the chapter.

COMPLETE THE COURSE IN ORDER

In the MBSR course there are specific reasons that certain meditations come before others. For example, the first few sessions include meditations with more guidance, because that's easier for beginners to do. Each session does not stand fully on its own. The sessions are built on the learning and development of the sessions before. In my experience, working through the program sequentially will make the course easier for you to follow and improve your understanding of mindfulness.

The next chapter offers a number of additional ideas for getting the most out of the program. Read on when you're ready.

THREE

Getting the Most Out
of Mindfulness-Based Stress Reduction

*The Chinese use two brushstrokes to write the word
"crisis." One brushstroke stands for danger; the other
for opportunity. In a crisis, be aware of the danger—
but recognize the opportunity.*
—JOHN F. KENNEDY

RANI WAS relentlessly rushing at work as she prepared for a big event.
She had lots of e-mails to get through each day, as well as phone calls
and long meetings. She'd just moved to a new house, and her husband
was away working on a project. She wanted to get everything done in
preparation for a vacation in California in a couple of weeks.

With too much to do and too little time, Rani's back started to hurt.
This was a familiar experience. Whenever she got too stressed, her back
acted up—probably due to the physical tension in her muscles. She knew
that if she didn't do something about it, things would get worse. In the
past, she'd been laid up for weeks with back pain.

She had done one of my MBSR programs a year ago and still had
the guided meditation audio but had somehow gotten out of the habit
of regular meditation. She decided to listen to the body scan meditation
every day before work. This immediately seemed to help ease the pain.
In the quiet of meditation, she also realized exercise could help and made
time to walk briskly and mindfully to the train station each morning.
She made sure to cut down on her multitasking and focused fully on one
task at a time.

The back pain began to melt away within a couple of weeks. She was
better enough to go on the vacation she'd planned and then return to
work refreshed. Since then, Rani has managed to keep up with the daily

mindfulness meditation practice. She realized how important the regular discipline was for her well-being.

The actual MBSR course is an 8-week commitment. If you're doing the full course, you commit to doing the home practice of 30 minutes a day for 8 weeks. If you're doing the mini-course, you need only about 10 minutes a day, which should be easier to fit into a busy schedule. After the 8 weeks, if you don't feel you've gained any benefit from the mindfulness, you can stop. There are, however, a number of ways to boost your chances of emerging from the program with significantly reduced stress.

The Importance of Daily Practice

Probably the most important thing you can do during the MBSR course is to do your best to practice mindfulness every day. Why is daily mindfulness practice so important? Because mindfulness is about training the brain. And if you want to rewire your brain, the key is repetition. Each time you repeat a process, the neural connections involved in that activity are strengthened. Learning mindfulness is like learning any new skill. Let's say you want to learn to ride a bike. If you try every day, even for just 10 minutes, you'll soon get the hang of it. And getting the hang of it simply means you're forming new neural pathways in your brain so the new skill becomes easier for you. Just as physical exercise is not something you do for a few weeks and stop if you want to be fit, mindfulness is a mental exercise that works through daily practice.

Take, for example, being aware of your breathing. Mindfulness of breath (described in Chapter 5) is one of the simplest and yet most powerful forms of meditation. When you first try this, you may find that your mind wanders a lot. You may feel very agitated. With daily practice, however, you can get better at it. At least you won't feel quite so agitated when your mind wanders. And your brain will become more mindful, which means you may begin to notice more about your surroundings and your own thoughts and emotions. You won't be on automatic pilot so often. The daily mindfulness practice has taught your brain to be more awake and conscious in the present moment, rather than just allowing your mind to wander all the time. Without a daily practice, your brain goes back to those old habits, which are simply the effect of your old neural pathways in your brain.

You may find the mindfulness practices easy and enjoyable. If so, great! But you may find yourself facing challenges when trying to instill mindfulness into your life.

> Mindfulness is simple in theory
> but can be challenging in practice.

Here are some of the challenges that have come up for my past participants:

- Finding time to practice
- Remembering to practice
- Overcoming resistance

And here are some tips for overcoming those challenges.

FINDING TIME TO PRACTICE

There are two main ways to apply mindfulness that you need to remember to practice every day during the course in this book:

- **Mindfulness meditations**—the daily meditation itself, which you make time to practice for either 10 minutes a day (mini-course) or 30 minutes a day (full course).

- **Everyday mindfulness**—being mindful in your routine activities such as brushing your teeth or walking to work, which encourages you to do one thing at a time and with full mindful attention.

Everyday mindfulness is a matter of remembering, rather than having the time. I'll say more about this later in the chapter.

The mindfulness meditations demand your time. As with anything worthwhile, you do need to find some time, even just a few minutes to reap the benefits of mindfulness. Here are some ways you could do this.

- **Schedule your mindfulness practice first thing in the morning.** I like to practice mindfulness as soon as I wake up. That way it's done and I can get on with the rest of my day. It also helps to set the tone for the day. Many of my students prefer to meditate first thing too.

If your morning is already full of activity, you could wake up earlier to carve out time to practice. This may seem like a drag, but the meditation could prove more deeply restful than your sleep.

- **Practice mindfulness when unoccupied during the day.** You probably have lots of short moments during the day when you're not fully engaged in a task—waiting for a train, sitting on a bus, waiting for a colleague to arrive at a meeting or for your child to finish playing in the park. These moments can easily be wasted, lost in thought. Instead, use them to practice a short mindfulness exercise.

For example, if you commute to work on a train, you may be able to do some of your meditations on that journey. One of my clients continues to practice all his meditations on his train ride to work and arrives fresh and energized.

- **Focus on your high-priority tasks.** Make an inventory of your daily activities. Label the activities as high, medium, and low priority. Just a few minutes away from any low-priority task can be used to practice mindfulness.

- **Make finding time a game.** Instead of thinking of meditation as a chore, see it as a game.

Take a few minutes to meditate while your computer starts up. Catch a mindful minute as you walk down the stairs. Be proud of yourself when you find 5 unexpected minutes to meditate—and tell others about it too. That will help remind you to keep an eye out for a few mindful minutes.

Reflection

What are you going to do to ensure you find time to practice your mindfulness? Jot down some possibilities in your journal as a reminder.

Finding a Mindfulness Buddy

If you're doing this mindfulness program without a teacher, one way to ensure you find time to do the practices is to acquire a mindfulness buddy. Someone who is experienced in mindfulness meditation would be a good choice. If you can find someone to meditate with, even if it's just once a week, that's going to help motivate you tremendously. But even if this person can't do the mindfulness practices with you, you can make yourself accountable to someone else by telling him or her about your commitment to complete this 8-week course. And when you start to doubt yourself, your mindfulness buddy can encourage you.

Your mindfulness buddy can be your partner, a son or daughter if one of them is old enough, or even one of your parents. Alternatively, one of your friends or a coach would make an ideal mindfulness buddy.

By the time you finish this chapter you will probably know what you need the most help with and how your mindfulness buddy could encourage you to stick to your commitment. But you can also offer the following guidelines.

A mindfulness buddy:

- Contacts you at least once a week.
- Asks you how your mindfulness practice is going.
- Encourages you to keep going in a positive way.
- Asks open-ended questions like "What happened this week in your mindfulness practice?" or "What aspects of the mindfulness do you find enjoyable or challenging?"
- Listens without judgment, especially without negative judgment.
- Meditates with you whenever possible.

REMEMBERING TO PRACTICE

One of the biggest challenges that my clients face is remembering to practice. They want to be aware, focused, and in the moment, but just keep forgetting! This is quite normal and very much part of the experience of learning mindfulness. In truth, no one is perfectly mindful—everyone forgets to be mindful and gets lost in daydreams, worries, and concerns at some point.

"I practiced the mindfulness audio together with my husband and young son after work, lying in our bed. They were so supportive. Even our dog joined in sometimes!"

The best way to remember to be mindful in your everyday life is to practice the mindfulness meditations. If you're willing to carve out some time to meditate every day, your brain will change and make you more likely to be present in your everyday life.

But how do you remember to practice your mindfulness meditation? Planning ahead is often the best way to remember to practice. Consider deciding where and when you are going to practice beforehand. If you plan each week of mindfulness meditation practice and make a commitment in your mind, you're more likely to be mindful. To increase the chances of sticking to the daily meditation even further, consider all the different things that could happen to prevent you from doing the practice and consider some ways of overcoming them.

You can choose to fill out the table on the facing page (also available to download and print from *www.guilford.com/alidina-materials*) to help you decide when and where you could do your daily meditations. These are the times of day you wish to do your meditation—it could be right after waking up every morning, just before breakfast, during your midmorning break, just before or after lunch, while you sit on the train to work or once you arrive home from work. You can choose whatever fits best in your schedule. Just don't pick a time when you feel sleepy.

Schedule for Mindfulness Meditation Practice

Day	When and where will you practice your mindfulness meditation?	What barriers do you foresee to meditating?	How will you overcome them?
Monday			
Tuesday			
Wednesday			
Thursday			
Friday			
Saturday			
Sunday			

From *The Mindful Way through Stress*. Copyright 2015 by The Guilford Press.

BEING CONSISTENT: OVERCOMING RESISTANCE

We all resist doing things we're "supposed to" do. Mindfulness can be like that too. It happens to me as well. I know I need to practice mindfulness because I'm highly aware of all the benefits, and yet I sometimes feel a certain resistance. You may also feel this resistance from time to time.

Mindfulness meditation practice may be a lovely, pleasant experience on some days but a pain on others. That doesn't mean mindfulness isn't working. To go back to the gym analogy, if you want to build up muscles, lifting up the weight is going to hurt. That doesn't mean you stop! "Ah, the gym thing isn't working," you may say. "Lifting those weights hurts—something must be wrong." That's almost the point. By working through the resistance, you discover a newfound strength. With mindfulness, practicing even though you feel annoyed or tired or agitated is working through an inner resistance. And although that may not be enjoyable, the long-term outcome will be worth it.

In my experience, the best way to deal with this inner resistance is by following these steps:

1. **Recognize that you feel a resistance** to do the mindfulness practice. Say the word "resistance" in your mind. This process of labeling helps to engage the more intelligent, wiser part of your brain.

2. **Identify what form that resistance takes.** Is it a thought like, "I can't be bothered to meditate!" or "I don't have time!" or "I don't feel like meditating!"? Or is it a feeling, such as a sensation in the pit of your stomach, a furrowing of your brow, or tightness in your chest? Where in your body do you feel the emotion?

3. **Now recognize that you're already practicing mindfulness!** By being aware of the resistance to practice, you're *being mindful*. You're noticing and acknowledging an experience in the present moment with a sense of curiosity.

4. You can develop this by seeing if you can **accept that resistance just as it is.** Be with the feeling or thought rather than fighting it. Be nice to yourself, using words like, "It's okay and natural to feel like this." Try to use a comforting tone of voice within your thoughts. Speak softly within your own mind, as if you're talking to someone you care about.

5. **Add to this experience a few deep breaths.** Feel your in and out breath, no matter what you're doing, such as washing the dishes, reading yet another e-mail, or watching TV. As you feel your breaths, **put a slight smile on your face**, recognizing and smiling at that familiar inner resistance and how you're being mindful of it.

Try this exercise when you feel some resistance to practicing mindfulness meditation, or whenever you feel resistance to do anything. Then write down in your journal what you noticed. What did you learn from this process?

A few months ago I started checking my phone in the morning as soon as I woke up. I was watching for a particular e-mail. But then, within a week or so, checking my phone first thing in the morning instead of meditating had become a habit. To counteract this habit, when I notice myself doing this, I continue to hold my phone in my hand and take a few deep breaths. I close my eyes and notice any resistance to meditate. I keep breathing. Then I usually feel the desire to meditate as stronger than the desire to use my phone. I sit up and do my meditation, knowing my e-mails can certainly wait another 20 minutes if they've been waiting all night. This is a nice way to let go of an unhelpful habit, notice resistance, and engage in meditation all at the same time!

Put Mindfulness on Your "To-Be" List

I don't wish mindfulness to be the cause of more stress for you. You have plenty of things that stress you out, I'm sure. Mindfulness is not another thing for your "to-do" list. Mindfulness is more than just a set of techniques that you need to integrate into your busy schedule. Yes, making time for mindfulness meditation is important, but it's more than that.

I meet many people who say, "Oh, I really *should* be meditating. It's so frustrating. I can't do it because. . . . " I can see that meditation is actually the cause of their stress. If this happens to you, I suggest you stop beating yourself up about it and just forget trying to meditate for a while. Yes, stop trying to meditate. Take a break from the relentless need to improve your life. Instead, just watch what's happening in your life, without the *should*s and *must*s. To really watch what's happening in your life and what thoughts and emotions you're going through is meditating—it's meditating on your own life, the most important meditation of all.

Mindfulness is a way of being. Mindfulness offers a way of working through that to-do list without frantically multitasking, panicking, or worrying. If mindfulness just sits on top of that list as another thing to check off and forget, you have something exciting to learn.

Mindfulness is a way of navigating through life knowing there's more to life than completing that to-do list. Life is far too mysterious to be limited to getting things done. It's about learning to take a break when you need it. It's about noticing the feeling of guilt or agitation when you do something nice for yourself and doing it anyway, knowing it's beneficial in the long run for you and those you care for. It's about doing nothing from time to time.

Think of mindfulness as underlying all your life experience, rather than another thing to do. See mindfulness as the soil from which you grow your life. Or as an anchor that you drop when it's time to stop the ship of your life. Just as your body needs air to breathe and food to eat, so your heart and mind need mindfulness and self-compassion to work harmoniously. This leads not only to a life with less stress but also to a life with greater joy.

There is more to mindfulness than just doing the practices, though. Studying and exploring concepts of mindfulness with others helps to keep the process exciting, fresh, and fun.

For example, if I wanted you to get enthusiastic about cooking, I wouldn't just tell you to start cooking. I'd give you a few good books on the subject, maybe a magazine, and get you to join a local class where you could learn more about cooking from others. With all these factors, your interest and skill in cooking would grow rapidly.

Think of mindfulness as being made up of three strands: mindfulness practice, studying mindfulness, and exploring mindfulness with other people.

- **Mindfulness practice.** This is the meditations and the everyday mindfulness exercises. Practices include expanding awareness meditation, body scan meditation, mindful movement such as yoga or tai chi, mindful walking, and even mindful conversations.

- **Studying about mindfulness.** This includes reading books on mindfulness or meditation in general and poetry about mindfulness, attending lectures or workshops, and listening to mindfulness talks online.

- **Exploring mindfulness with others.** This can be with a friend, a mindfulness group, a mindful workshop, or even online. My mindful online community is at *www.facebook.com/shamashalidina* or on twitter *@shamashalidina*. Feel free to say hello or to ask me a question on there—I'm happy to help.

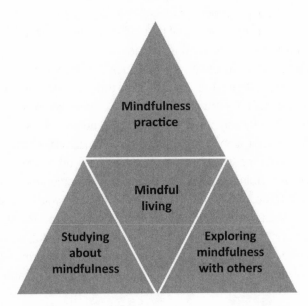

Of the three processes, mindfulness practice is the most important. That is the process that rewires your brain to be more mindful and resilient to stress. But the other two paths can help you remain consistent and overcome resistance to the practice of mindfulness.

(TIP) If you don't have time to study mindfulness or explore mindfulness with others, just stick with doing the mindfulness practice you learn in this book. To continue the cooking analogy, although reading more cookbooks and talking to friends who are skilled cooks can be helpful, it's not essential. Just practicing cooking is the important bit.

Keeping a Record of Your Practice

I'd recommend you keep a record of your mindfulness practices and reflections in a journal. Keeping a record of your experiences of practicing mindfulness has several benefits, especially if you're working through this book on your own. They are:

• **Directly reducing your stress.** By writing down your thoughts and feelings, you are able to take a step back, to decenter, from them. This is an important aspect of mindfulness. The act of writing down your thoughts and feelings has a stress-reducing effect in itself. Journaling has been shown in several studies to reduce stress.

• **Identifying patterns.** By regularly recording your experiences in a journal, you're able to notice patterns in your behavior. For example, when you practice mindful exercises in the morning, you may have less stressful experiences during the day, whereas afternoon meditations make you feel sleepy. Mindfulness is about observing yourself and others so that you can gain insight—the writing process is a mindfulness practice in itself, giving you insight into patterns of behavior that could reduce your stress.

• **Discovering solutions.** Writing down your experiences helps you work out solutions to your stressful problems. Thoughts have a habit of circling around and around in your head. Getting them down on paper reduces the spiraling thoughts and gives you a clearer perspective about the situation.

One of my clients, who had a stressful time in the recent economic downturn, kept a regular record of his mindfulness practice. Whenever he came to see me, he handed over his worksheets showing me what arose for him that week. During the first week, he seemed to be enjoying the

> "Journaling is something that I hadn't tried before. I found it surprisingly relaxing and therapeutic. I use it whenever I have time or am feeling stressed. I do a short mindful exercise and then start writing!"

meditations and exercises. But after a few weeks, the number of meditations started to reduce. I asked him why. He realized that as soon as his stress levels went up, when he had an important meeting coming up, he would stop meditating—just when he needed it most! He redressed this balance and felt much better for it. It may seem obvious to you reading this now, but if you don't write down records of your practice, you can miss the most clear patterns and links.

Research Corner: Journal Away Your Stress

Philip Ullrich, MA, and Susan Lutgendorf, PhD, of the University of Iowa, researched the effect of journaling on stress levels for 122 college students. They asked one group to journal about their thoughts and emotions of stressful events, one group to just focus on the emotions of stressful events, and one group to write about general news events. They discovered the students who were asked to write about their thoughts and emotions developed a greater awareness of the positive aspects of the stressful events. The group that just focused on writing about the negative emotions seemed to feel worse by the end of the study.

So, Are You Ready?

Now that you know what to expect from the course in this book and how to get the most out of it, how do you feel? Excited? Hesitant? Anxious?

You can never be 100% prepared for this or any other course. You can only do your best and see what happens. The perfect time will probably never arrive. As long as you are interested in trying the course, and aren't currently in the middle of a major life change, give mindfulness a proper try. You never know what you'll discover until you commit to the mindful exercises. And if you slip with your mindfulness practice once in a while, that's okay. These things happen. How many times do you think you fell over when learning to walk? To make mistakes is inherent in any learning process. So have a go and see what happens. And remember, there are lots of people who will be willing to support and encourage you along the way if you ask. Asking for help when you need it is a sign of strength, not weakness. Good luck!

FOUR

Week 1

There's More Right with You Than Wrong with You

What lies behind us and what lies ahead of us are tiny matters compared to what lives within us.
—HENRY DAVID THOREAU

INTENTIONS

✦ *To begin exploring what mindfulness actually is.*

✦ *To experience the mindful body scan meditation to gently train your attention, to learn about the nature of your mind to wander, and to become more familiar with bodily sensations.*

✦ *To understand the concept of automatic pilot through some mindful eating.*

WHEN CHENG first started learning mindfulness, he was suffering from chronic fatigue syndrome. He was unhappy, and life was not going well. His relationship with his wife was in tatters, and he felt completely inadequate and guilty about how he struggled to make enough money to support his two daughters. He felt so stressed that he couldn't even put it into words.

His doctor suggested a course in MBSR, and he didn't understand what mindfulness was but was willing to try anything. When he first meditated in class, he found it so difficult. His mind was all over the place. He felt he wasn't getting anywhere. It felt like a complete waste of time. His meditations ended with feelings of tearful anxiety. Sometimes the meditation left him feeling angry too. His teacher encouraged him to continue, telling him that the mix of emotions rising to the surface of

51

his awareness was actually a good thing and a part of letting go of inner emotions that he had trapped within him. Cheng felt this was true, and a deep longing for inner calm encouraged him to persevere despite the challenges.

Fast-forward a few years later, and Cheng's life has totally changed. His chronic fatigue syndrome is gone. He occasionally sees his doctor for a checkup, but that's it. He has been meditating diligently since the MBSR course and loves it with a passion. High levels of stress truly are a thing of the past for him. His family life seems a thousand times better, and he is able to live a full life with his kids and wife. Cheng is grateful for every day that he lives. Although he can't be sure that the meditation alone caused this transformation, he certainly feels it was central to his healing process. Needless to say, he's a big fan of mindfulness for reducing stress and healing.

You may or may not be suffering from the huge challenges that Cheng did when he first started MBSR. But I hope this story gives you a sense of the potential of meditation. And although you may not heal dramatically from an ailment like Cheng did, you are likely to find a healthier way of coping with your stressful challenges, whatever they may be, with greater mindfulness.

So I'd like to warmly welcome you on this journey toward living your life more mindfully. If you like what you discover, you're encouraged to continue to practice indefinitely into the future, in any way that fits with your lifestyle and needs.

In this chapter, you begin the first part of the MBSR course. Remember, you have two routes available to you and two ways to go through the chapter:

- You can follow either the full or the mini-course.
- You can begin reading and trying each mindfulness exercise as it comes up (preferable but not essential) or you can read through the chapter first, to get a feel for what it's all about, and then go back and try the mindfulness exercises.

Discover: A Miracle Is Taking Place

You may be reading this book and considering learning mindfulness for a range of different reasons. Perhaps you or a loved one suffers from stress due to a health condition such has heart disease, cancer, chronic pain, depression, or anxiety. Maybe the stress is linked to your circumstances, such as an overly demanding job, exams, family circumstances, or living space.

With high levels of stress and disease comes a feeling of being broken, hurt, or damaged. However, you're still breathing. And if you're breathing, we're exploring the following possibility:

> There's more right with you than wrong with you, no
> matter what you're going through.

Your body is achieving something incredible. It's nourishing itself with a finely balanced level of oxygen and breathing out excess, unwanted gases. No matter how much of a failure or how broken you feel, you can breathe. And as long as breathing is happening, a miracle is taking place, and it's right under your nose. (Sorry for that breathtaking pun.)

Your body is a piece of engineering that no scientist can come close to fully understanding, even today. Each of your senses has evolved to work so efficiently, accurately, and sensitively, you are unlikely to fully value them until they stop working. And your brain is considered the most complex piece of engineering in the known universe.

Mindfulness is an invitation. An invitation to turn inward. An invitation to discover the pattern and wisdom of your thoughts and emotions. To explore the range of physical sensation that you may be so quick to judge. To make the time and space to stop, for just a moment, and see with fresh eyes. It's a radical act of waking up. You may find this inner journey a little scary because you're not sure of what you'll find in there. But you don't need to leap into the deep end. Just start by dipping your toe in and, step by step, discover the most precious treasures that were so much closer than you ever imagined.

So let's begin together. Dip your toe in with a short yet powerful mindfulness exercise.

PRACTICE: Opening Awareness Meditation

Audio track 2: 10 minutes.

Here's a short exercise to give you the flavor of mindfulness. Give the exercise a try and see what happens. Spend about 10 minutes doing the Opening Awareness Meditation—the exact timing is not important at all. Make a note of your feeling of stress before and after this exercise, just out of curiosity. In mindfulness, the idea is to be curious about your stress rather than fixated on lowering it.

1. Sit in a comfortable posture so you can be relatively still. Take a few deep **breaths**. Feel the sensation of each breath as you inhale and exhale.

2. Notice the **colors**, shapes, and patterns that are entering your eyes, without judging them as likes or dislikes. You may think "carpet," "ant," or "I've never noticed that pattern before." Whatever thought arises, acknowledge it and turn your attention back to just looking and noticing the colors.

3. **Now** close your eyes if you wish and turn your attention to sounds. Become aware of sounds entering your ears. Allow the sounds to be registered just as they are. Again, you don't have to purposefully identify the sound—just listen to the quality of the sound itself.

4. Move your attention to **sensations within your body**. You don't need to find pleasant or strong sensations—whatever sensation you notice in the body is absolutely fine. See if you can feel the sensations in your body as a whole.

5. When you're ready, shift your attention to your **emotions**, if that's okay with you. Become aware of how you're feeling, right now. Does the feeling stay the same or change from one breath to the next? Can you notice where the emotion rests in your body?

6. Finally, become aware of your **thoughts**. What thoughts are arising in your mind in this moment? What are you thinking? Just notice the thoughts passing by, like clouds that float across the sky. If you get caught up in a train of thought, that's okay. Just step back again when you can.

7. Now let go of focusing your attention on anything in particular. Just notice whatever is predominant in your awareness, without making any choices. Practice **choiceless awareness**. It may be sounds, thoughts, your bodily sensation, or something else. Just step back and observe your moment-by-moment experience. You don't need to do this perfectly—whatever happens is absolutely fine.

8. Bring this exercise to a close by taking a few deep breaths and gently opening your eyes and noticing your surroundings again.

Congratulations. That may have been your first experience of mindfulness. It is also quite special because it includes all the different forms of mindfulness meditation at once.

In some ways, the whole course and everything you'll learn is contained in the Opening Awareness Meditation. This is because it includes an awareness of your breath, body, all your senses, and the inner world of thoughts, emotions, and even awareness itself. There's nothing else you can be mindful of, so you covered them all in that exercise!

(TIP) If you ever feel stressed and aren't sure of what meditation to do, just do the Opening Awareness Meditation.

Reflection

1. What did you notice in this short exercise? Consider your thoughts, feelings, sensations, and anything else.
2. What did you find easy and/or difficult about the exercise?
3. Do you find yourself judging or criticizing yourself for not performing well in the experimental practice? Can you let that go, as you are a beginner just starting this mindfulness course?

Discover: Your Best Self

When you're under stress, you're much more likely to focus on what's going wrong. This is the way your brain works when stressed. Your brain looks for threats and usually overestimates them. Recall the last time you saw someone stressed out: was the person calm when something went wrong, or did she overestimate the negatives, creating a mountain out of a molehill?

I think it's helpful to begin this course in a positive frame of mind. You may be going through considerable difficulties and not want to even consider anything positive. But I gently encourage you to have a little go at it.

I've been reading a book called *Winning without Losing*. It was co-authored by Jordan Milne, who talks about ways of being successful in your work but making time for family, friends, and whatever else you love. He recalls one sentence that his mother repeated to him every day. She used to say to him every morning, while looking him in the eye, just before he set off for school:

"Look for the good things."

She then gave him a warm smile and watched him walk to school until he was out of sight. This sentence is now ingrained in his brain, and he's always looking for the good things in life, even when things go wrong. If you want to take a shot at looking for the good things in your life right now, try the following exercise.

EXERCISE: **What Is Your Best Self?**

Answer the following questions and try coming up with at least one answer for each. Resist turning your answers into negatives by following what you say with "but . . . " That negates any positives that you've written down. Be honest and realistic and see what arises. Enter your answers in your journal if you like.

This exercise is not intended to get you to see life through rose-colored glasses. But if you have too much stress in your life, you may be wearing dark glasses. As you're reading this book, you have a choice—a choice to see things in a different light.

1. What are you like when you are at your best?
2. What are you like when you're relaxed?
3. What are you grateful for in your life right now?
4. What makes you happy, either now or in the past?
5. What gets you excited?
6. What's going well in your life right now?

By doing this exercise, you're shifting your perspective on your own life. And this is one of the keys to managing stress. You'll learn more about this in Chapter 5.

Discover: Why Are You _Really_ Here? It Matters

One of the first things I do when I'm running an MBSR group is to go around and ask the participants to share their names and, if they're willing, to share *what* they hope to get from mindfulness.

Following is an exercise you can do to help you explore your innermost desires for doing the program. This is important, because knowing your own motivation helps to deepen your discipline—you're more likely to wake up those few minutes early to meditate when you are clear in your mind as to what you hope to get from the course.

In addition, being clear about what you hope to get from mindfulness illuminates your *intentions*. And your intention is intimately related to the quality of your mindfulness practice.

Dr. Shauno Shapiro, Associate Professor of Psychology at Santa Clara University, together with colleagues, has suggested that mindfulness is built on three dimensions: intention, attitude, and attention.

1. **Intention** is about why you're doing the mindfulness in the first place. What do you hope to get from it? What benefit would it have on others around you?
2. **Attitude** is how you cultivate that mindfulness—attitudes like being nonjudgmental, curious, and accepting. Your attitude is like your viewpoint or frame of mind when practicing mindfulness.
3. **Attention** is what you focus on. Your attention develops through repeated practice, built on your intentions and attitudes.

You will learn more about attention and attitudes as you work through this course. The following ocean visualization is one way of clarifying your intentions.

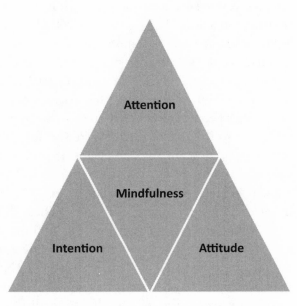

EXERCISE: Uncovering Your Intention—
Mindful Ocean Visualization

Audio track 3: 10 minutes.

This is a mindful visualization that takes about 10 minutes. You don't
have to be good at visualization to be able to do this. The idea is to just
try your best and see what happens. The purpose of the visualization is
to reflect a little deeper about what you hope to get out of learning and
practicing mindfulness. You may think you already know, and that's fine,
but by doing this exercise you never know—you may discover something
new.

1. **Get comfortable.** Find a relaxed posture for this exercise. Get
   comfortable on your favorite sofa or chair. You could even lie
   down if you want. Just try not to fall asleep if you can!
2. **Think of a beautiful and peaceful beach.** It could be a beach
   you've visited in the past, or you can make one up, or you could
   combine the two. At this point you may be filled with indeci-
   sion. "Which beach shall I choose? I must choose the perfect
   beach!" Choose any nice beach—the important point is not
   the perfect beach, but to choose one beach and stick with it for
   the duration of the exercise if you can.
3. **Imagine you're sitting on the beach**, near the water. You could
   be sitting on a deck chair or on the sand, whatever you prefer.
4. **Notice what you see.** Become aware of what you are able to see
   as you sit by the side of the ocean. Notice the color of the sky.
   Is it sunny or cloudy? Is the sun rising or setting? Is the horizon
   clear? What can you see along the beach? Is it deserted, or are
   there other people around? Are there palm trees or other trees
   behind or to the side of where you're sitting? Can you see any
   cliff edges? Are there any birds flying around, near or far? You
   don't need to be able to visualize it perfectly. Just notice what
   you can see without trying too hard.
5. **Be aware of what you can hear.** Can you hear the sound of the
   ocean as the waves come gently rolling in? Take time to hear it
   if you can. What about the sound of the breeze against the trees
   or the birds as they call out? Enjoy the sounds. Notice whether
   you find it easier to see or hear the experience within you.
6. **Notice the scent.** You may be able to smell the ocean or just

a familiar scent of being on the beach. What's it like to notice that scent? Rest your attention on the scent of your experience for a few moments.

7. **Be aware of any taste in your mouth.** Perhaps the taste of the saltiness of the water or maybe no taste at all.

8. **Be mindful of how your body feels.** How does your physical body feel as you sit peacefully by the side of this beautiful ocean? Does it feel relaxed, tense, or somewhere in between? Notice the light touch of the breeze against your face, arms, hands, or feet. Is the gentle breeze warm or cool?

9. **Pick up a pebble.** As you sit on the beach, you notice a pebble. This pebble represents the question, "What do I hope to get from mindfulness?" You ask yourself the question as you pick up the pebble. While you hold the pebble in your hand, you once again reflect on the question, "What do I hope to get from mindfulness?" without forcing any answers.

10. **Throw the pebble.** You look at the pebble and look out at the ocean. You are able to throw the pebble into the ocean, and you do so. You're able to see the pebble move in slow motion. It rises up high and gradually falls into the ocean. The pebble creates some ripples and begins to sink into the water.

11. **You can follow the pebble and reflect as it sinks.** You are able to see this beautiful pebble as it slowly sinks deeper and deeper into the ocean. The deeper the pebble sinks into the ocean, the deeper you reflect within your own being, "What do I hope to get from mindfulness?"

12. **Reflect.** As the pebble sinks deeper toward the ocean floor, you reflect deeper within yourself, asking "What do I really, *really* hope to get from practicing mindfulness?" You don't need to force any answers. You may get a word, phrase, image, feeling, or sensation. Or you may not get anything at all. That's okay. Just see if you can reflect on the question and accept whatever happens. Keep gently bringing your attention back to the visualization if your mind wanders off, noticing what your mind was thinking about.

13. **Ocean floor.** Eventually your pebble comes to rest on the ocean bed. You are somehow able to see the pebble resting on the ocean floor. You reflect back on your experience.

14. **Gently ending the visualization.** When you're ready, you can come back to sitting on the beach, looking out at the ocean. You notice the scenery and leave it behind for now, but know

that you can come back to it anytime you wish. You now return from this inner world to the outer world but can bring with you any insights you wish to bring.

TIP You can use this as a daily mindfulness practice if you want. You can just use the imagery and leave out the reflection part if you prefer.

Here's an example of what happened to Jane, a student of mine, when she did this exercise. When Jane joined a mindfulness group, she was suffering from anxiety. That's why she'd signed up to do the class. She'd had some anxiety her whole life, but now, with the frantic nature of work, it was getting unbearable. She thought the only reason she was doing the course was to get rid of the anxiety. But after doing this mindful visualization, the word *clarity* kept arising for her. She realized that running away from the anxiety was a fear-based desire that led to confusion. What she really wanted in her heart was to move toward greater clarity in her life. That's why she was doing the course. This put her in a good starting place to begin her mindful journey within.

What was your experience of the visualization like? What do you want from mindfulness—deeply in your heart?

Explore your experience in the following reflection. If you didn't really engage well with the practice, try again later on today or some other time this week.

Reflection

Write down what you noticed at each of the following stages. Remember, there's no right or wrong—whatever experience you had is correct.

- Looking out at the ocean
- Listening
- Scent
- Taste
- Touch—how your body felt
- Experience of pebble dropping into the ocean
- Effect of reflecting on the question, "What do I hope to get from practicing mindfulness?"
- Any other reflections on your overall experience

PROCESSING YOUR EXPERIENCE WITH THE VISUALIZATION

The idea of this mindful visualization is to see whether it helps you discover something deeper within yourself about your motivation for practicing mindfulness. You may discover that you wish to practice mindfulness for:

- Greater clarity
- A deeper sense of peace
- More calm
- Better focus
- A deeper sense of spirituality or religion
- More enjoyment in life
- Happiness

However, it may not be any of these.

It doesn't matter if you can't come up with the reason at the moment. By practicing mindfulness, your intentions will become clearer. Mindfulness is about accepting the outcome of your efforts rather than fighting with your present-moment experience. So bring to it a lighthearted attitude and an open mind if you can.

If you did discover your deep intention for practicing mindfulness, you could find an object, painting, or photo to represent this discovery. For example, if you wish to gain a sense of calm through the practice of mindfulness, you may place a picture of a beautifully still and crystal-clear lake surrounded by gorgeous mountains up on your bedroom wall. Then, each time you see the image, you'll be reminded of your deep intention. My clients have used pictures of their loved ones at work to remind them to be mindful there too—a great idea. With mindfulness, you'll probably discover that remembering to be mindful is the tricky part; any reminder is helpful.

Discover: Mindfulness Is Not Simply Relaxation

Mindfulness is not just a relaxation exercise. This is an important point to understand. **Relaxation is certainly a desirable side effect of mindfulness,** but relaxation may or may not arise in any one mindfulness exercise. Relaxation is about easing the tension in your muscles and lowering your heart rate. You can relax by taking a hot bath, by doing deep breathing exercises, or by allowing yourself just to daydream.

The intention of mindfulness is not simply relaxation. And there's a good reason for this. If your goal is to relax, you begin to look for that outcome.

Every time you don't achieve relaxation, your mind can start racing with thoughts like, "Why am I not relaxing? I can't relax. I wish my mind would just shut up!" and so on. Making relaxation or a calm mind into a goal can increase stress levels.

Mindfulness works by releasing habitual ways of thinking and reacting to the world around you. Your mind is always creating automatic ways of dealing with life, and those habitual patterns are old, and sometimes negative, unhelpful, and cause stress.

For example, let's say you want your son to mow the lawn. He just wants to watch television. Your habitual automatic thoughts may start saying, "Why is he so lazy? He should do more in the house!" Your heart starts beating faster, and you feel angry and start an argument rather than reasoning with him. Your stress levels rise.

Mindfulness takes a different approach. Mindfulness is about developing greater present-moment awareness. In the preceding example, you may pause before reacting, noticing your rising anger. You take a few mindful breaths and think about the most effective way to motivate your son. You may also remember that he has had a busy day or is watching his favorite TV program of the week. You can see how this process of mindful living has nothing to do with just relaxation.

By practicing mindfulness meditation, you're not just trying to relax either. You learn not to *react* to whatever experience arises within you, and this gets translated to the outside world. You learn to stop automatically reacting to challenging people, situations, and circumstances. Instead, you take your time to choose and *respond* more wisely, using the lens of mindfulness rather than past habits. In this way, your stress reduces.

Research Corner: Want to Relax?
Then Don't <u>Try</u> to Relax

In 2007, Shamini Jain of UCSD, Shauna Shapiro of Santa Clara University, and colleagues compared mindfulness meditation to relaxation training. They found both approaches beneficial in reducing stress and increasing positive mood. The interesting finding was that mindfulness meditators reduced cyclical negative thoughts (rumination), which relaxation didn't seem to do. Rumination deepens the grooves of negative thinking in your brain and also doesn't solve the problem you're faced with. And rumination is linked to anxiety and depression. So mindfulness seems to be a great way to help you reduce stress by decreasing your ruminative thinking patterns.

Through long-term practice, mindfulness leads to lower levels of stress, but in any given mindfulness practice it's about cultivating a kind, warm, caring awareness rather than just trying to relieve muscle tension or calm your mind.

> Mindfulness is not just a relaxation exercise. Mindfulness reduces stress by teaching you to respond consciously rather than react automatically to challenging thoughts, emotions, bodily sensations, or life situations.

EXERCISE: Mindfully Eating an Apple

Audio track 4: 10 minutes.

Here's a simple exercise that I'd recommend you to try out with a bite-sized piece of apple. To do this, you just need to sit down and reduce any potential distractions for the next 10 minutes or so. If you don't have an apple, you can use any small piece of food—experiment with raisins, bananas, chocolate, or even a marshmallow!

1. Begin by noticing what the apple actually looks like. Notice the color of the skin and the flesh. Explore the patterns in the skin and the subtle variations in color and the indentations. How does the light reflect off the apple? How smooth or rough does this piece of apple feel? What else can you notice as you continue to look at the apple? And what judgment comes to mind—thoughts about liking and disliking? Be as curious as you can.

2. Now close your eyes, if that's okay, and become aware of the sense of touch as you hold the apple. What does it weigh? How does it actually feel to have the apple in your hand? What is its temperature? Does it feel soft and delicate or quite firm? Do the muscles in your hands or arms feel tense or relaxed as you hold it? Take your time as you do this.

3. While keeping your eyes closed, *slowly* bring your apple toward your nose. Notice at what point you're able to actually pick up the scent of the apple. What does it smell like? Is the scent strong or subtle? Does it cause salivation as you smell it? Do you find yourself liking or disliking the scent?

4. Keep your eyes closed, allowing your arm to move downward and

rest for a few moments. Then, slowly and attentively, bring the apple toward your mouth. Notice whether any salivation is happening. Touch the apple gently against your lips to feel the sensation of that. Then place the piece inside your mouth. Be aware of what this feels like. Slowly place the apple piece between two teeth and notice which teeth you chose. Do you always chew with those teeth? Then slowly take your first bite into the apple. Connect with any sounds, tastes, and smells. What's the experience like? How does the flavor of the apple spread around your mouth? How does the texture of the apple change as you chew it? Continue chewing as slowly as you can, experiencing the apple as it gets broken down and swallowed.

5. Eventually, once you've finished eating the apple, notice any sense of an aftertaste in your mouth. Become aware of how your body feels.

VARIATION: If you find it difficult to focus in this practice, try labeling your experience. Say to yourself "picking up the apple," "green color," "feels cold," "smells sweet and fresh," and so on. Labeling experiences in your mind can help sharpen your focus.

Reflection

Now answer the following questions:

1. How was this experience of eating an apple?
2. How was it different from your normal experience of eating?
3. What did you like or dislike about the experience?
4. Why do you think this is not the normal way you experience eating?
5. How can you bring a greater element of mindful eating into your life?

Discover: Automatic Pilot

Mindful eating is a great exercise to show how often you eat without really tasting your food—and what happens when you stop to eat more consciously.

You notice tastes, flavors, and experiences you may never have been aware of before.

You're probably too busy to eat each meal as slowly as that. But perhaps you could reduce the multitasking you do when you sit down to eat? And what about other activities? Do you walk to work automatically, lost in your own world of thoughts, or do you notice the other people, the trees, the sky? And what about your interactions with your children, partner, or friends? Is that another habitual process, or are you conscious of their behavior, their body language, tone of voice, and what they're saying to you?

There are certain problems with living in an automatic way that lead to higher levels of stress:

1. You have **thoughts** popping into your head that may be causing you stress. For example, you may be thinking a particular project needs to be done perfectly because that's what you've always done. However, this is both impossible and unrealistic for the time frame you have available. So, unconscious, automatic thoughts can cause you stress.
2. You may be dealing with your **emotions** automatically. For example, you're feeling a bit nervous about your next date or about the fact that you don't even have a date. Instead of reassuring yourself, or talking to a friend about it, you may begin to fight with the emotion or deny it, leading the anxiety to grow unnecessarily out of control.

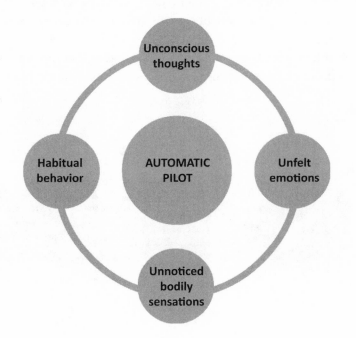

3. You may react to **bodily sensations** automatically. Every time your body feels tired, you may start to criticize yourself for being unhealthy or not looking after yourself. Or you don't even notice the tension in your shoulders or jaw until it's so painful that you have to stop. Taking earlier action, such as a short mindful break when you initially notice bodily tension, would reduce your stress.

4. Your **behavior** may lead to greater levels of stress. For example, whenever you're driving and someone cuts in front of you, you immediately get angry and start shouting and cursing. This makes you feel more stressed before you've even gotten to work or to school to pick up your child. You're on autopilot, and your stress levels are rising.

So, in all these different ways, you're living automatically, and these habitual tendencies are operating all the time.

Mindfulness is about giving yourself a choice. When you have choices, rather than automatically **reacting** to life with its challenges, you **respond** wisely. I use the word *reacting* to mean an automatic knee-jerk-type action or thought. I use the word *response* to mean more reflective, thoughtful, and conscious choices that you make. You'll learn more about how to do this as you go on with this course. For now, in this session, you just need to understand what automatic pilot is and how to identify when you're operating on automatic and when you're more conscious and mindful.

In the diagram below, you can see how living automatically and responding in a habitual way leaves you no choice when faced with life's challenges. And without choice, your thoughts, words, and actions could lead to higher levels of stress.

Mindful living leads to conscious, wise choices and restoration of balance. The diagram on the facing page shows a more mindful approach to

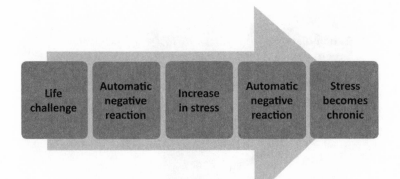

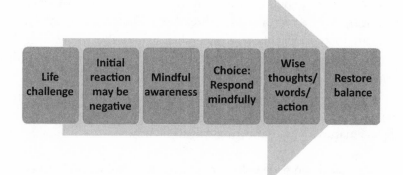

living. As you are faced with a life challenge such as a demanding job or an angry partner, by being more mindful you create space in your mind to make a choice. That choice can lead to wise decisions and therefore higher levels of well-being and lower levels of stress.

As Viktor Frankl, author of the inspiring book called *Man's Search for Meaning,* famously said:

> "Between stimulus and response there is a space. In
> that space is our power to choose our response. In our
> response lies our growth and our freedom."

Mindfulness is about finding that space and choosing your response.

EXERCISE: How Unmindful Can We Be?

To show you just how unmindful our brains can be in everyday life, check out this amusing video: *www.shamashalidina.com.*

PRACTICE: Mindful Belly Breathing

Audio track 5: 10 minutes.

This is a nice simple exercise for switching off your stress response. If you've been suffering from stress or anxiety for some time, chances are you breathe in a shallow way. One easy way to start easing your stress is to learn how to do deep belly breathing. Once you get the hang of it, you can do it at any time you remember. Eventually it may even become a habit for you to breathe more deeply, using your belly. This is likely to lead to deeper levels of relaxation for you.

Have you ever seen a baby breathing? The baby's belly usually expands on the inhalation and contracts on the exhalation. Belly breathing is a natural and comforting way to breathe.

1. Lie down on the floor, mat, carpet, or bed. Close your eyes if you wish. Place your feet on the floor with your knees bent.
2. Notice how stressed you're feeling. Assign a rating of 1–10 (10 for the highest stress) to your current stress level if you want.
3. Loosen any tight clothing, especially around your waist and neck. This ensures your breathing is not restricted.
4. Begin by just noticing the feeling of your breathing for about a minute.
5. Place one hand gently on your belly, in your navel area. Place your other hand on your chest.
6. Now as you naturally breathe in and out, notice which hand is moving: is it the hand on your belly or the one on your chest?
7. If your belly is rising and falling, and not your chest, you're already doing belly breathing. Continue to feel your breathing in the area of your belly for the next few minutes.
8. If you find your chest is rising and falling and not your belly, your breathing has some potential for improvement and, with that, a reduction in your feeling of stress. Simply see if you can get your belly to rise as you breathe in and not your chest. And when you breathe out, see if you can feel your belly dropping down, rather than your chest.
9. Try rubbing your hands together to warm them and gently massaging your belly area. Notice any feeling of relaxation around the belly area.
10. If this doesn't work for you, take a deep breath, and as you breathe out, gently apply pressure to your belly as if you're pushing the air out of your lungs. Then, on your next in-breath, you may find yourself drawing air much more deeply into your lungs and doing some belly breathing.
11. Continue to practice for 5–10 minutes. If you feel dizzy at any point, just go back to your normal, natural rate of breathing for a while, until you feel better.

12. Notice how stressed you feel on a scale of 1–10 again. Do you feel more or less stressed? Remember, please don't think you must feel more relaxed—just be curious and notice what's happening.

You can practice this exercise at any time of day or night. It's a nice exercise to do before you go to sleep and just after you wake up. And you can do the practice in a seated posture when at work or home. You can even try it while standing or walking. Belly breathing is also an exercise you can purposely engage in, whenever you feel anxious or tense.

Reflection

What did you discover about your breathing? What effect did the mindful belly breathing have on your feeling of stress?

Tales of Wisdom:
Live in the Moment for Stress-Less Living

I was recently in San Diego to give a talk on mindfulness at a conference. I had a couple of spare days in town after the conference, and was told that I should visit an aircraft carrier, which had been turned into a museum. So, together with a friend, I parked my rental car in the parking lot and went onto the aircraft carrier. The size of the carrier was amazing. We spent several hours walking all over and taking pictures. At the end of my visit, I reached for my pocket but couldn't find my car keys. We went to the lost property office, but they didn't have them either. I retraced my steps to the sleeping quarters, the deck, even checked on the actual planes that were on the carrier—but no luck. I'd lost the keys! And we had to catch our flight back to London the next day. All our bags and clothes were inside this rental car. Then I noticed a couple of sneaky thoughts in my head: "What if someone finds the keys and steals the car? How can I fly home without my passport?" But I caught these thoughts just in time, and smiled. I decided there's no point worrying about this—it won't help me find the keys. Instead, I asked where the nearest nice restaurant was, and we walked over to have lunch, overlooking the beautiful Pacific

Ocean. We soon began to laugh—of all the places to lose the keys, an aircraft carrier. It looked like one of the biggest ships in the world! After staying present, smiling and enjoying our sandwiches and fruit juice, I called up the lost property office. Good news! Someone had found the keys and had handed them in.

This ended up being one of the best stories of the trip. Just goes to show, when you're in the present moment, you can stop worries from sneaking up on you, and let them go. Even if we didn't find the keys, we could have called the rental company and gotten new keys. And if the car was stolen, it's possible to get new passports. For these everyday problems, there's often a solution if you pause and reflect for a few moments.

PRACTICE: Body Scan Meditation

Audio track 6: 10 minutes.

Audio track 7: 30 minutes.

Now you're going to learn your first, main meditation. It's called the body scan. The course starts with the body scan meditation for several reasons. First, because the meditation is normally done lying down, you don't need to worry about managing any pain in your back or other parts of your body. You can just let the ground support the weight of your body. Second, the practice involves quite a lot of guidance, so you are not left on your own with long periods of silence. As a beginner, this is usually quite helpful.

How does this body scan meditation reduce stress?

- When stress levels rise, your body often tenses, or an emotion is felt in your body. The purpose of the body scan is to train your mind to focus your attention on your body sensations. Awareness of your body will help you notice when your stress levels rise so you can take suitable action, rather than allowing it to spiral out of control.
- The body scan meditation may also relax your muscles, one of the side effects of mindfulness. Many people report the process to be relaxing after long-term practice. Some of my clients call it "a massage from the inside out."

- Habitual, automatic negative thoughts are one of the causes of stress. Through the body scan, you learn to notice and let go of these thoughts and shift your attention to your body. This is one way of controlling your stress. The body scan teaches you to notice your body, without judgment.
- You learn that by being mindful of stress and the feelings of anxiety within your body, you can process the emotion without a need to react to your stress in any way.
- You may not like or respect your body. That can be stressful. The body scan teaches you to be friends with your body—you're going to be together for life, so you may as well be friends! The body scan meditation can help create a more positive relationship between you and your body.

This mindfulness practice is designed to last 10 minutes if you're doing the mini-course or 30 minutes for the full course. The exercise involves methodically resting and moving your attention from one body part to the next and noticing what sensations are present with a sense of non-judgmental curiosity.

The drawing below is the typical posture used in the body scan meditation. The posture is called the corpse pose. The practice is a great, easy way to relieve stress, lower blood pressure, and encourage relaxation and can help with insomnia, tiredness, and headaches.

(TIPS) Ask a friend to check the alignment of your head in this pose. It's common for heads to be tilted to one side; your friend can help by carefully and *very* gently lifting your head and realigning so it is equidistant between your shoulders, with your nose pointing toward the ceiling.

If you have lower-back issues or it just feels more comfortable, you can raise your knees toward the ceiling and put your feet flat on the floor or use any posture you prefer, including sitting on a relaxed chair.

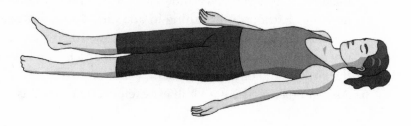

Script for Full Body Scan Meditation

To do the mini-body scan, simply spend less time on each body part.

1. Begin this meditation by finding a time and place that's right for you. Turn off any potential distractions and ensure your room is not too hot or cold for you.

2. Lie down on the floor, mat, or firm mattress with your legs straight and your feet falling slightly away from each other.

3. Begin by noticing your breathing. The breath is such an essential part of being alive and yet is so often forgotten. Notice the whole cycle of the in-breath and out-breath, without trying to judge or control it if possible. Just be aware of it from moment to moment. If you wish, feel your breathing down in your belly, your lower abdomen. If you can't feel any sensation there, you could try placing your hands gently on your belly if you wish.

4. As you practice this body scan, if at any time you feel overwhelmed by sensations or emotions, remember you can shift your attention back to your breath if that feels comforting for you. You can think of your breath as a refuge from any sensations that seem too much for you at this time. That is probably the kindest and most helpful thing you can do at that time and is totally fine.

5. Now, when you're ready, shift your attention from your breathing, down your body, down your left leg, and all the way down to the big toe in your left foot. Feel any sensation that's present for you. If you can't feel anything, just feel the lack of sensation—that's perfectly fine. Then move your attention to your little toe and the toes in between. Then the sole of the left foot and the heel; the sensation of the heel touching the floor. Now feel your left ankle and any sensation there. And around to the upper part of your left foot with all its bone and muscles and tendons inside. Feel the left foot as a whole now. To help develop your awareness, you may like to play with the idea that your breath can go down and into and out of your left foot. Imagine or feel your breathing carrying a mindful awareness into your left foot. If breathing in and out of your feet doesn't mean anything to you, just let it go. It's fine to do that. Then, when you're ready, let the sensations in your left foot fade into the background of your awareness.

6. As you practice this mindfulness exercise, your mind is going

to get distracted and lost in other thoughts. That's totally normal and nothing to get disheartened about. Mindfulness is not about banning thoughts.

7. In this way, move your mindful awareness into your lower left leg, upper left leg, then start with your right foot and move all the way up your right leg.

8. Let your attention rest in the area of your hips, pelvis, buttocks, and all the sensitive organs in this part of your body. Be aware of how the sensations shift and change from breath to breath. Again, imagine your breath being able to go into and out of this part of your body if you find it helpful. Then, when you're ready, allow this part of your body to fade into the background of your awareness.

9. Continue to work through your body in this mindful way, up to your lower torso. Be aware of and sensitive to the rising and falling of your belly and any emotions that may be present in that area of your body.

10. Move up to the upper part of your torso. Feel the contact of your back against the surface you are resting on. Feel your chest area and the movement of your rib cage as you breathe in and as you breathe out. You may be able to feel your heart beating. Get in touch with any emotional signals or sensations in your emotional heart, if that feels okay for you to do. Imagine or feel your breathing going into each body part to increase your sense of awareness. Feel sensations with an attitude of affection or kindness, the way you may look at something precious or someone or something you love. If possible, reflect on how fortunate you are for the parts of your body that are working okay, that are ensuring that in this very moment you are not only alive but also present and mindful of them.

11. Continuing to move through your body with a kindly awareness, feel and accept the sensations in your shoulders, including any tensions that don't release. Then down your arms into your hands and fingers. Take a moment to feel the intricate sensations present in the tips of your fingers.

12. Then move your awareness gently up through your neck, including the back of your neck, your throat, and your voice box and into your face. Feel the surface skin of the face and the muscles underneath. Begin with the forehead and move down into eyebrows, eyes, cheeks, lips, mouth, teeth, tongue, jaw, sides of face,

Dealing with a Wild Mind

Almost all the clients I see say their mind just can't focus in the mindfulness practice, and they feel they're doing something wrong. The fact is, your mind is going to wander off into other thoughts; it happens to the most experienced practitioners. That's just something you have to accept. These are some of the things that you can expect to happen as you practice mindfulness meditation:

- You find you were thinking about other things for most of the meditation.

- You felt like you were doing nothing at all even though you wanted to focus on the meditation.

- You feel as if your mind became more active, having done the meditation.

- You didn't enjoy the meditation because of all of your thoughts.

These are all quite normal experiences. The key is not to ban thoughts, but to accept them as part and parcel of mindfulness practice. Mindfulness is about being aware of the thoughts, and then gently guiding your attention back to the focus point.

Think of your point of focus like a puppy. As you take a puppy for a walk along a path, she will naturally get interested in someone off the path. Her attention will get captured and she'll wander off. Once you notice, you don't jerk your puppy back—that would hurt her. Instead, you gently pull the lead back to the path. Then before long, the puppy will wander off again. That's okay; you just guide her back to the path. In the same way, expect your mind to wander off, and gently, kindly, affectionately guide your attention back to the point of focus. You may even like to congratulate yourself for noticing that your mind has drifted off, rather than criticizing yourself for a wandering mind. The key to mindfulness is plenty of patience and trust in the process.

ears. Then feel the weight of your head against the surface it rests on. See if you can go inside your head to feel the presence of your brain. Notice how it feels. And last, but not least, the top of your head.

13. Notice what it feels like now that you've mindfully scanned through your entire body. Rest for a few moments, whatever that means for you.

14. Now, this is an optional extra process that some people find helpful: Imagine that your breath can sweep up and down your body. As you breathe in, you can imagine your breath sweeps up your body, and as you breathe out, your breath sweeps back down again. You can get a sense of your breath feeding each of the living cells in your body with nourishing and wholesome oxygen. This may seem a bit strange to you, but just play with the idea and visualization or feeling and see what happens for a few minutes.

15. Now, letting go of all effort to practice mindfulness, just rest in your own inner sense of presence, of aliveness. Rest in your innate sense of *being*. You have nothing else you have to do, nowhere else to go, and nothing you need to achieve. Simply being.

16. Finish by gently congratulating yourself for having practiced this mindfulness meditation. It doesn't actually matter how it went—what's important is you made the time to practice. Each practice, no matter how you judge it, is beneficial.

VARIATION: If you keep falling asleep when you do the body scan, don't worry about it. You can try keeping your eyes open, or try sitting up on a chair.

GOING DEEPER: At the end of the body scan meditation, continue to practice for a further 15 minutes or so. Rest in open awareness like at the end of the expanding awareness meditation (see Chapter 8).

Remember: No matter what your experience was, keep practicing. You may have fallen asleep, felt more anxious, found it boring, discovered you couldn't concentrate, or just felt uncomfortable. Just try to make yourself as comfortable as possible next time and keep practicing. Know that the human mind is very wild, and if it takes you in directions you didn't plan on while trying to meditate, welcome to the club—and see the box on the facing page.

The body scan meditation is not an easy practice for many people, especially at the beginning. Persevere with the exercise in the week to come with an open mind and just keep noticing what happens. And if you found the process easy, that's great!

Reflection

1. What bodily sensations did you notice in the body scan most strongly? Which parts of your body had no sensation?
2. Did you notice your mind wandering? What sort of thoughts did you have?
3. How did the experience feel for you? What emotions arose and passed away during the process?

Discover: Thinking of Problems Differently

Consider whatever is causing your distress at the moment. The death of a loved one, a challenging work situation, or being under financial pressure is not easy to handle. In this mindfulness course, we are not asking you to run away or deny that challenge at all. But you are encouraged to explore the possibility of seeing it in a different way.

Mindfulness helps you see things differently because:

- You're practicing the skill of stepping back and seeing the big picture.
- You're learning to pay attention to other things rather than your problem.

Take a stab at trying to solve some of these puzzles, which require "thinking outside the box." See if you can think about your own problem in the same way and notice what happens, if anything.

1. What could this represent?

   TO   CH
     U

2. A woman pushes her car up to a hotel and immediately realizes she's bankrupt. Why is that?

3. The nine-dot puzzle:

   ● ● ●

   ● ● ●

   ● ● ●

Look at the nine dots arranged on the facing page. Your challenge is to draw four straight lines through all the dots, without taking your pencil off the paper. Each line begins where the last line ends. You can start anywhere. Give it a try.

Give it some time and don't give up too easily. You could try a bit of mindful breathing before you start, or halfway through if you find yourself getting frustrated.

See page 82 for the answer, but give yourself at least 5 minutes to try to solve it, and most important, observe what strategy you adopt to solve the problems.

There are three main things to learn from these puzzles, which you may be able to apply to the challenges in your own life.

1. WORK SMARTER, NOT JUST HARDER

If you keep trying the same strategy or approach, you won't necessarily get an answer. You need to let go of current ideas and take a step back. More effort may just lead to frustration rather than a solution. Stress arises when you keep trying the same strategies and don't get the result you're looking for. Use mindfulness to take a step back and see things in the opposite way. Many people talk about working smarter rather than harder, but mindfulness gives you a practical way of achieving a smarter mindset.

For example, I was really struggling with a deadline for a presentation I was preparing. Trying to fit that in with my other role of mindfulness coach and having lots of meetings, I couldn't get my presentation done. It felt stressful to be juggling so many balls. I did a short mindfulness exercise and decided to look for a more radical solution. The answer came: to completely rearrange my schedule. By taking a week off from meetings and working on my presentation full-time, I finished the preparation and felt much more energized and excited.

2. EXPLORE THE BOUNDARIES

Are the boundaries of the solution something you have created artificially in your mind? What would happen if you changed those limits? Are the boundaries based on your perception, or are they reality? Be clear about the rules you've set yourself. By being mindful of the limits you've placed on yourself or the situation, you can release stress.

When I first began teaching meditation, I didn't think I was good at all. That thought had an impact on my teaching. After listening to the positive feedback from my students and letting go of this stress-inducing thought, I began to relax and enjoy teaching meditation much more. Now I've discovered a much more enjoyable attitude to teaching: I just make sure that I'm having fun as I teach! If the students enjoy and benefit from the class, that's a bonus. That's a much better way to live and the students seem to love it.

3. LOOK BEYOND THE LIMITS OF THE PROBLEM

If you're not clear about the problem, no matter how hard you try, you won't come to a solution. Try to think of your problem in different ways.

One of my colleagues was really stressed about her financial situation. She was struggling to pay all her bills even though she owned several businesses. She saw her problem as the need to pay the bills and felt stuck for not having enough money. Then, after talking to a friend, she realized her problem was actually being too attached to her businesses. She sold one, had more cash available, and felt freer. With a calmer and more creative mind, her other businesses began to flourish. The problem was not lack of money but of attachment.

EXERCISE: Finding a New Way to See a Problem as a Challenge

Now consider one of your problems that you're willing to explore and see it as a challenge to be solved in a different way. Consider the tips above and write down what your challenge is (use your journal or jot some notes here) and any new or unique ways of coming up with solutions.

Problem/challenge:

Different ways of seeing the challenge:

Possible unique solutions:

Mindfulness Meditation FAQs

Q: Am I doing it right? How do I know if I'm doing the meditation correctly?

A: As long as you're doing the practice, you're doing it right. All that you need to learn will arise in the meditation practice—you just need to learn to trust in yourself. So whenever you have the thought, "What if I'm not doing this right?" just say to yourself "thinking," and bring your mind back to wherever you were focusing your attention. How did you learn to walk as a child? You just go for it. It's the same with meditation.

Q: I felt restless in the meditation. How can I stop that?

A: Perhaps cut down on your caffeine intake or other stimulants during the day. And try to do your daily activities with more mindfulness; that may reduce the feeling of restlessness in the meditation. Try going for a short, slow walk, noticing the feeling of your breath. A few deep, slow breaths at the beginning of the meditation can also help to switch on your relaxation response and calm your restlessness. But beyond that, see if you can "work through" the restlessness. This means to allow the restlessness to be there as you meditate. Try noticing which part of your body feels most restless and feel the physical sensation together with your breathing. Be interested in the feeling rather than trying to work out how to get rid of the feeling. It will pass.

Q: I couldn't focus on my body. My mind was wandering all over the place. What's wrong?

A: Nothing. The very fact that you know that your mind was wandering is mindfulness. Not knowing that your mind was wandering is mindlessness. So first, remember that you have been mindful. Second, in meditation, as in the rest of your life, your mind wanders. It's the way your mind works. Expect your mind to wander, and when you notice, bring your attention back. That whole process *is* mindfulness. Nobody has ever done a full body scan meditation or any other meditation without the mind wandering—it's impossible and not the aim of the practice. Try smiling when you notice your mind has wandered; many of my students love this practice.

Q: I felt really relaxed. Is that okay?

A: Yes, absolutely! Just don't expect relaxation every time. Sometimes it comes; sometimes it doesn't. You just need to bring a gentle awareness to whatever you're focusing on. If you feel relaxed, enjoy the feeling of relaxation.

Q: I didn't find it relaxing at all. Why is that?

A: Relaxation may or may not happen. Avoid making relaxation a goal.

Instead, just try to be aware of your bodily sensations or breathing as best you can. The benefits arise from that and from bringing your attention back again and again when your mind wanders.

Home Experiments: Week 1

Here are the mindfulness experiments for this week. The table at the end of this section spells out what you need to try, depending on whether you're doing the mini or full course.

Body Scan

Try practicing the body scan every day at a time that suits you. You'll probably find it easier to make use of the audio to help guide you in the practice.

Mindful Belly Breathing

This is an additional activity for those doing the full course. You simply need to take 5–10 minutes, sit in a chair or on a meditation cushion on the floor, and feel the sensation of your breath. You can feel your breath around your nose, chest, belly, or wherever else you prefer. Expect your mind to drift to other thoughts, and when you notice, guide your attention back to your breath.

Mindful Booster

As you go through your week, you'll be forgiven for not being mindful all the time—it's so easy to forget. One way to creatively counteract this automatic tendency for habitual living is to use a mindful booster, an activity that you do as mindfully as possible to help raise your level of mindful awareness.

This week's mindful booster is taking a shower (or bath) mindfully. To do this, you take a few conscious breaths before your shower and set an intention to be mindful. You probably have a particular shower routine—try mixing your routine up. If you normally wash your hair first, wash your hair last. Changing your routine will increase your mindful awareness. Be mindful by connecting with your senses in each moment. There's the sound of the water splashing against your skin, the scent of the soap, the warmth of the water, and the physical sensation as the water hits your body. It can be very enjoyable! As with any other meditation, when your mind wanders, bring your attention back to the present moment.

Reflection

Jot down your experience of the mindfulness home experiments every day. You may like to use these questions to help you reflect on your experience. Taking time to reflect in this way helps you grow in wisdom and discover your own personal habits and attitudes.

- What effect did the practice have on your thoughts, feelings, and bodily sensations?
- How motivated did you feel to practice before and during the process?
- What did you discover through the mindfulness exercise?
- What could you change or adapt next time you practice, if anything?

Week 1

Day	Mini-Course	Full Course
1	Mini-body scan Mindful booster	Body scan Mindful belly breathing Mindful booster
2	Mini-body scan Mindful booster	Body scan Mindful belly breathing Mindful booster
3	Mini-body scan Mindful booster	Body scan Mindful belly breathing Mindful booster
4	Mini-body scan Mindful booster	Body scan Mindful belly breathing Mindful booster

Day	Mini-Course	Full Course
5	Mini-body scan Mindful booster	Body scan Mindful belly breathing Mindful booster
6	Mini-body scan Mindful booster	Body scan Mindful belly breathing Mindful booster

Answers to the questions:

1. "You're out of touch."

2. She's playing the board game "Monopoly."

3.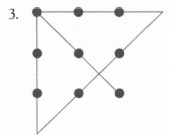

Week 2

From Automatic Reacting to Creative Responding

A busy person is not someone who has lots to do.
A busy person is someone who does too many things at
the same time.

—AJAHN BRAHM

INTENTIONS

✦ *To explore the role of personal responsibility and interpretation in stress.*

✦ *To learn the mindful pause.*

✦ *To try some new ways of dealing with stressful thoughts.*

ANASTASIA WAS a successful banker in the city with a stressful job and a busy family life. She loved her husband and two children dearly. In recent years, she hadn't enjoyed her job at the corporate bank, but it paid the bills—and they had a lot of bills. Her mind was often quite fuzzy, as if she was looking through a smoke screen all the time. With all her responsibilities, she felt like she was juggling lots of balls. Multitasking was an everyday occurrence. Constant busyness was her way of living. She had worked long hours as far back as she could remember. Almost everything seemed to run habitually, on automatic pilot.

On a Monday morning, and without warning, Anastasia experienced her first panic attack. This wasn't a butterflies-in-the-stomach-before-an-interview type of feeling—this was more like being on the edge of a cliff, as if her life was threatened. She thought she was having a heart attack and felt extremely shaken up. Anastasia was rushed to the hospital, but the tests came back negative; her heart was fine.

Her doctor explained that the panic attack was linked to her high levels of stress and recommended that she do an MBSR course to learn to use mindfulness to manage her stress levels. Anastasia was willing to try anything to avoid a recurrence of that awful feeling, so she quickly signed up.

The experience of the meditations in the MBSR course was extremely challenging for Anastasia at first. She couldn't feel much in her body at all. And then she started to feel anxious in the meditations and begin crying for no apparent reason. Was crying normal? she asked. Her teacher reassured her that people do sometimes cry at some point in meditation and it was perfectly normal. He had a kindness about him and offered encouragement and support, so she persevered. Anastasia really wanted this to work.

Within weeks Anastasia found the mindfulness meditations deeply nourishing for her in some ways. The anxiety began to diminish, and she discovered a feeling of peace she hadn't felt for a very long time. Meditation was like coming home to herself after a long, arduous journey away. She was starting to feel more complete and whole. She felt like she'd be running at full speed on a treadmill and had exhausted herself. There were now moments in the day when she could slow down or stop that treadmill without fear that things would fall apart.

Fast-forward several years, Anastasia practices mindfulness regularly and feels fully rejuvenated from the daily meditation practice. She's able to enjoy a much happier family life. But the biggest impact is the way she deals with challenges in life. Rather than her old, negative pattern of constantly worrying, she is calmer and more reflective.

This chapter explores how to go from automatically reacting to people and situations in life to consciously responding and making wise choices about the best way to deal with any given situation, just as Anastasia learned to do in her life.

In mindfulness, **reacting** means to not notice the choice you have made. To immediately go from facing a difficult situation or thoughts to taking automatic, habitual reflex action. This could be arguing, shouting, thinking negatively again and again, or any number of different actions. Reactions tend to be negative, because you don't give the wise part of your brain time to work properly.

Responding means to make a conscious choice about your thoughts, words, and actions in any given circumstance. For example, noticing that you're judging yourself as stupid and letting it go. Being aware that you're feeling sad and not fighting or running away from the emotion. Or when a colleague says something hurtful, taking a few moments to reply rather than starting a heated exchange.

Mindfulness is about responding to life's challenges
with wisdom and self-compassion.

Going from habitually reacting to consciously responding to life's difficulties isn't easy. But the principles and shifts of mind required are not as difficult as you may think. With a little bit of patience and determination, you can learn to take small steps toward mindfulness. And small steps are all that is required of you—nothing more and nothing less.

Personal Responsibility: Getting Your Stress Under Control

You may think of responsibilities as increasing your level of stress. The typical image of someone who is under too much stress is someone who has taken on too many responsibilities. And this may be true. You can take on too much work—more than you feel you can handle.

But self-responsibility is different. I'm talking about being responsible for your *response* to your stress. If you just blame outer circumstances for your stress, you may feel a little better in the short term but are probably setting yourself up for higher levels of stress in the future by not taking appropriate action. Although taking responsibility for your stress may feel like a burden at first, it's actually the first step to reducing stress in your life. Anastasia eventually took responsibility for her stress and used mindfulness to respond in a more healing way to her illness, family, and working life.

You can see the effect of lack of self-responsibility when dealing with habits. For example, let's say you have a habit of biting your nails. If you think nail biting is just part of your personality or due to your parents also biting their nails, there's no chance that you can reduce or stop your habit of biting your nails, even if you want to. Not until you think, "I'm responsible. I'm doing the nail biting, and I am determined to stop it," do you have a chance. The same goes for your response to your stressors—you need to trust in your own inner ability to manage them better.

There are some things that you can't control. If, for example, you are faced with a major stressor such as the serious illness or death of a loved one, your stress levels will shoot up—you can't easily change that. However, you can slowly begin to manage the way you respond to that stress. You need to allow yourself to go through the natural process of grieving, sadness, and anger before you come to terms with the loss or change in circumstances. Mindfulness offers you the space to do that. You can learn to manage the stress itself with wisdom, awareness, and self-compassion.

Taking responsibility for your own stress doesn't mean you need to judge or condemn yourself for feeling stressed. Quite the opposite. Self-responsibility offers hope, giving you ways to use mindfulness to recognize when your stress is high, and discover new and powerful ways of responding to that stress. Mindfulness encourages you to be kind to yourself, to treat yourself as you would treat a friend who was under stress.

Here are some mindful ways to shift toward taking control of your stress:

• **Remembering that you always have a choice in life**. If you don't have a choice about the external situation that's causing you stress, you can still choose your attitude. There are even examples of people in Nazi concentration camps who used this approach to deal with the stress by remembering that they could still control their attitude.

• **Practicing mindfulness meditation.** This will show you how your thoughts affect your feelings and bodily sensations and vice versa. You therefore see that much of stress is an internal experience.

• **Watching out for thoughts like "I have no choice" or "There's nothing I can do about this."** Step back from these thoughts rather than entertaining or believing them to be true.

Reflection

Think back to a time when you were experiencing some stress but felt in control. What was your attitude toward the stress? What happens when you apply that attitude toward the stress in your current situation?

Interpretation and Stress

One major part of controlling your response to stress is to control your interpretations of events.

Not every potentially stressful event—your angry boss, your whining child, or your inbox full of e-mails, to name a few—is felt as stress by all people (or even by each individual all the time). You could interpret your angry boss as "He's just in a bad mood today," your child's whining as a passing phase—"He'll get over it"—and your inbox as "That's just the way things are in modern life. I'll sort it out when I have more time tomorrow morning."

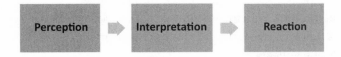

In truth, the emergence of stress is a complex interaction of many factors, but your interpretation of the stressor is a very important one. Your interpretation of a stressor determines whether your stress response is engaged, which may be felt as anxiety or tension or in some other way. Consider the following example.

I was watching a series of comedy clips the other day. In one clip, someone put a moving toy snake on the floor in a hallway. When the unsuspecting owner opened her front door, she saw the toy snake and jumped in fright. Her cheeky family members immediately burst out laughing, and within seconds her fear was turned into laughter as she realized the snake was just a toy. This seemingly silly example can explain why some people suffer from high levels of stress whereas others don't.

When the lady first perceived the image of a snake, she thought it was real. So she thought, "Oh my goodness, a snake!" or perhaps even stronger words. With that thought, her stress response was switched on. Within a second, stress hormones were released to make her heart beat faster and muscles tense up.

If she continued to believe that the toy was a snake, she would continue to feel stressed and under threat. The same is true for your stressors. As long as you interpret them as threatening, you'll continue to feel stressed.

This story illustrates the three steps that produce the stress response:

1. **Perception** of situation—see a wriggly thing on the floor.
2. **Interpretation** of situation—thought: "It's a snake!"
3. **Reaction** to the situation—stress response switched on, heart races, jump with fright, tense up.

The key point here is that your interpretation is required before you find yourself stressed.

You interpret a situation as threatening before your
stress response is switched on.

If the person who saw the snake actually worked at the zoo with snakes all day, she probably wouldn't be scared at all. Interpretation makes all the difference.

Optical illusions are a great example of how your brain interprets what it experiences. Look at the central circle in the diagrams below.

Which one appears bigger?

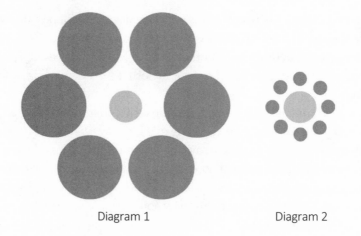

Diagram 1   Diagram 2

Most people say the central circle in the second diagram looks bigger. But if you measure it, you'll find they are both exactly the same size. Why were you deceived?

The illusion works because of the circles that surround the central circle. In Diagram 1, the circle is small relative to the surrounding circles, so it looks small. In Diagram 2, the surrounding circles are smaller, so it looks *relatively* bigger. Your brain uses this comparison to assume the central circle in Diagram 1 is smaller than in Diagram 2.

Your stressor is not *directly* the cause of your stress. The level of stress you experience is actually linked to how much you believe your thoughts about the stressor. I don't mean to diminish the very real feeling of stress you are experiencing. Nor am I saying that your stressful life is a product of your thinking alone. But interpretation plays a bit part.

Shakespeare takes this to an extreme, as he states in *Hamlet*:

"For there is nothing either good or bad,
but thinking makes it so."

Now that you know that interpretation can lie at the root of stress, your next questions may be, "Why do I interpret situations in this way? Why do I see things as threatening and end up stressing myself out unnecessarily?" This is actually the nature of the human mind, and intimately links to human evolution, as I explain below.

THE NEGATIVITY BIAS: YOU'RE WIRED TO FOCUS ON THE NEGATIVE

If you find yourself being more pessimistic than optimistic, it's because your brain is wired that way, as it is for most humans. This theory is called the negativity bias—the tendency to give more attention and weight to negative experiences and information.

The reason is thought to be evolutionary. Consider life in early human history. Some humans probably took risks and wandered around the jungle hunting for food. They didn't worry too much about getting eaten by the local tiger. Other humans took minimal risks. They worried more. They got stressed more easily, and any suspicious movement in the bushes would send them running, energized by their stress response. They probably would have felt more stressed and anxious. Which one was more likely to survive and therefore able to have children? Obviously, the more cautious ones. The humans who took fewer risks and remembered the dangers lurking outside survived. They reproduced, and their genes got passed on to the next generation.

> "Before mindfulness, I never knew my thoughts affected my feelings. And I didn't know that I could step back from my thoughts. I just reacted to life and lived on autopilot. Now I know I have a choice. Why didn't they teach me this at school?!"

That's why, in the earlier example of the snake, the lady jumped up with fright almost instantly—her mind immediately registered the negative, that it was a snake, and reacted accordingly. This is a built-in survival mechanism called the fight-or-flight response. (In Week 4, you'll read more about the physiological response involved in this primal alarm system in the brain.)

The following examples may show your tendency to focus naturally on the negative news:

- Your car doesn't start in the morning, and you tell all your friends that evening about that fact. You don't mention the sunny weather, the fact that you didn't have a car accident, or that your colleagues were friendly to you that day.

- You receive bad service at a restaurant. You don't consider that the food was fine, that the view of the lake beside the restaurant was stunning, or that your health was excellent that day. Noticing the positive aspects of the restaurant experience would take conscious effort.

- You feel lonely and lethargic today. You focus on your low mood rather than the fact that you're spending time in the countryside later that week, that your children are perky and cheerful, or that you have time for a long and refreshing walk if you choose to take one.

- You're much more likely to pick up a newspaper with a negative head-line rather than a positive one. Bad news hijacks your attention and sells more. Interestingly, this wasn't the case on April 18, 1930. The BBC announced, "There is nothing newsworthy worth broadcasting," and played piano music instead! This would be unheard of nowadays and gives a little insight into why our current levels of stress may be higher than they used to be: a constant stream of mostly negative news, available on TV and online 24 hours a day.

All these typical examples just show how easy it is to focus on the nega-tive experiences rather than positive ones. And constant focusing on the negative can cause an excessive buildup of stress.

Research Corner: Three Tricks Your Brain Plays on You

Neuroscientist Rick Hanson says there are three ways your brain tricks you to ensure your stress levels are heightened, which doesn't improve the quality of your life in modern society:

- Overestimating threats

- Underestimating opportunities

- Underestimating your ability to manage opportunities

These tendencies often increase your stress levels unnecessarily. You can use mindfulness to manage them by:

- Being mindful when you feel threatened. Ask yourself to consider or write down all the things that are actually going well at the moment. This helps to shift things to the positive.

- Being mindful of the actual risk of taking the opportunity in front of you. For example, getting on a plane may feel scary, but in reality it's one of the safest modes of transport.

- Noticing when you think, "I can't do it," and questioning yourself. Is that actually true? Is it most likely your negativity bias at work? Think about times when you thought you couldn't achieve something and you did. For example, if you're going for an interview, think about past interviews that were successful.

DANCING MINDFULLY WITH YOUR BRAIN'S INTERPRETATIONS

So your brain has a tendency to focus on the negative due to the negativity bias—but can you do anything about it?

Practicing mindfulness meditation has been shown to shift the negativity bias, rewiring people's brains after even just a few weeks of daily practice. And the shifts from more negative, fear-based thinking to more holistic, open, and optimistic ways of meeting daily life can be seen in brain scans.

In addition to mindfulness, here are five main areas you can work on. Let's say you're finding it very stressful to sit in a traffic jam for the purpose of illustration:

1. **Flex your attentional muscles to reinterpret the stressor.** Mindfulness trains your brain to be able to move your attention from one place to another, instead of just focusing on worries. For example, rather than seeing the traffic jam as making you late, you can see it as a chance to listen to your favorite music, to do some mindful breathing, or to listen to an audiobook. To do this, you need to be mindful that you're seeing the situation negatively and then consciously shift attention to more positive outcomes.

2. **Practice gratitude.** Think about all the things that are going well in your life. Use mindfulness to really become aware of what you're grateful for. So in a traffic jam, you could consider five things that are going really well in your life and the reasons that they make you feel good. And you could even send a text or e-mail, or call, once you arrive at your destination to thank whomever you were thinking of. Expressing gratitude is even more powerful than just thinking about it.

3. **See the big picture.** Although your stressor is causing you anguish at the moment, will it make a difference in the long run? With the traffic jam example, will this really matter in the next week, month, or year? Does this really matter in the great scheme of things? One of the key aspects of mindfulness is the ability to step back and put things in perspective. Most things in life are never as bad as they seem; that's worth remembering.

4. **Be kind to yourself instead of self-enforcing perfection.** If you set very high standards for yourself, you're setting yourself up to fail. Continuing the example of the traffic jam, notice whether you always want to be on time. You can aim to be on time, but being on time 100% is impossible. The mindful way of dealing with perfectionism requires you to see that each present moment is the only way it could be, right now. Focusing your attention on the present moment rather than trying to create an idealized future helps to slowly release perfectionism. Another tip is to try to achieve 80%

of perfection in any task and notice that the world doesn't end when your outcome isn't perfect.

5. **Mind your language.** Be mindful of the language you use in your thoughts. Words like *always, never, should,* and *must* are signs that you're thinking in extreme ways that could be feeding your stress. Step back from those thoughts and see them as thoughts rather than facts. Or ask yourself questions like "Is that true? Am I *always* late?" or "Why *should* I rush to get there on time and risk my safety and that of others on the road?" More on this in Chapter 8.

Reflection

These reflections are helpful whenever you feel overwhelmed by stress. Try them out now and use them again whenever you feel overly stressed.

Consider a current source of stress for you at the moment—not your biggest source of stress, but something significant. This gives you an opportunity to practice interpreting stressors differently. Enter it in your journal if you like, along with the answers to these questions:

1. What's going well for you at the moment? (This could be simply that you have a roof over your head or have had enough to eat today.)
2. How can you see the stressor differently? Can you see the stressor as a challenge? If so, does this challenge have any benefits?
3. Will this stressor be such a concern in a few months' time? Or a few years' time?
4. Are you setting very high standards for yourself? Can you aim for 80% perfection instead? Consider doing a simple task less than perfectly and practice being with the uncomfortable emotion rather than acting on it. The emotion will pass.

Remember: Some stressors may seem too big for this type of viewpoint. If the particular stressor for you is divorce or a loved one's terminal illness, or perhaps you yourself are threatened in this way, this is of course very challenging. In these circumstances, kindness toward yourself, giving yourself space to grieve, and plenty of rest are all important. You need to find someone with empathy to listen and support you. And you may find that mini-mindfulness

---

Research Corner: Posttraumatic Growth

Stephen Joseph is a pioneering psychologist at the University of Nottingham who has spent the last 20 years working with trauma survivors. He has discovered something incredible. For *most* people, traumatic events like illness, divorce, assault, bereavement, accidents, natural disasters, and even terrorism can lead to positive changes in the long run. In other words, traumatic events act as catalysts to personal growth! This doesn't mean that the trauma didn't cause stress, difficulties, nightmares, and other challenging experiences. What it does show is that the experience can often lead to growth, rather than a disorder.

Joseph's book, *What Doesn't Kill Us: The New Psychology of Post-Traumatic Growth,* includes a range of examples of people who grew in wisdom in the aftermath of disaster. He says hundreds of studies confirm that 30–70% of people experience a positive outcome in the aftermath of trauma—posttraumatic growth is almost the norm. People report that their relationships become deeper, they feel more mature and wise, and they often reprioritize their lives for what's truly important to them, rather than chasing status and wealth as they may have previously.

Posttraumatic growth is an excellent example of how many people reinterpret stressors to help reduce their stress and increase their resilience for future stressors they may face.

---

meditations help you get through each day, moment by moment. Changing your interpretation is not appropriate when a major stressor is fresh in your mind, but perhaps, in time, you can consider such an approach.

EXERCISE: Reacting and Responding to Your Own Thoughts

Here's an exercise to show you how your brain interprets situations and how that interpretation can lead to stress if you react to it. Take a few moments to imagine the following scenario happened to you. Be aware of how you'd think and feel in the situation. Take your time as you read this:

Imagine you're in a local café . . . You sit down . . . The waiter comes over to take your order . . . You order a cup of coffee and a croissant . . . The waiter takes the order . . . You wait to get your drink and snack . . . 5 minutes pass . . . 10 minutes pass . . . still no sign of the order . . . 15 minutes pass and you don't receive your order . . . there's no sign of the waiter . . .

What thoughts pop into your mind in that situation?

How do you feel (e.g., sad, angry, calm, annoyed, not bothered, scared, bored)?

When I do this exercise with different people, I get different answers. But the situation is the same: a waiter doesn't deliver an order. Here are some possible thoughts (interpretations) and feelings.

Interpretation

"This waiter hates me. This always happens to me. I should be more assertive. This isn't going to be a good day."

Feeling

Sad. Dejected.

Interpretation

"The waiter's probably really busy. It's not an easy job being a waiter. I think I'll go and remind him of my order."

Feeling

Calm.

Interpretation

"Typical waiter. He's pathetic. So lazy. I'm gonna have a real go at him. Let me find him."

Feeling

Anger.

Notice the pattern between the interpretation and the feeling? When you blame yourself for the situation, the result is a low mood and dejection. When you blame the other person, the result is anger and frustration. And when you don't place the blame on anyone, but just circumstances, the feeling is neutral, or perhaps concern.

This exercise shows that thoughts play a part in shaping your feelings. Or more accurately, **the thoughts you believe to be true** affect your feelings. In the past, psychologists encouraged people to change their thinking to be more realistic. But a new, mindful approach is emerging to deal with difficult emotions. You just need to train your brain to see the thoughts as just that, thoughts or interpretations. Mindfulness exercises and meditations train your brain to respond to your thoughts and emotions rather than react automatically.

> "After I got burned out due to stress, I started reading self-help books. I didn't even know self-help books existed! I realized that my thoughts played a big part in the stress I experienced. I'm far more mindful of my thoughts now. I practice a short mindful exercise as soon as I begin to get too stressed out."

Here's another little experiment you can do. Try thinking, "I can walk through walls." Say that to yourself a few times. Have the thought in your head. Do you believe it to be true? Of course not. And so you're not going to even try walking through a wall. In the same way, when you notice your thoughts as just an interpretation rather than a fact, you learn to give those thoughts less importance because you don't *believe* them to be true.

> Stress is not caused just by thoughts, but the thoughts that *you believe to be true.*

Reflection

The next time you feel stressed, notice what's causing the stress. Then notice what thoughts are causing the stress.

Write down the stress-inducing thoughts. Are these thoughts absolute fact, or are they an interpretation?

(TIP) Body posture and movement do affect thinking and interpretation. Experiment with sitting up straight, going for a brisk walk, holding a smile on your face for 20 seconds, or taking 10 deep, mindful breaths.

Now see if you can interpret the situation differently. What effect did these little techniques have?

PRACTICE: The Mindful Pause Meditation

Audio track 8: About 2 minutes.

This week you're going to learn an important mini-meditation called the mindful pause. This is a meditation that I recommend you practice daily from now on.

The purpose of the mindful pause is:

- **To turn off automatic pilot mode.** This is the habitual mode your brain defaults to. This mini-meditation switches that off so you can be more conscious and create a change in the way you react to your experiences.
- **To become more aware of your thought patterns.** This mini-meditation helps you stop in your everyday life and become aware of your thoughts. Destructive thought patterns could be the cause of your stress. You can notice and step back from them using this mindful exercise.
- **To become aware of your stress.** By stopping to do the mini-meditation, you notice what your stress level is like. You can then begin to work out what's causing the stress. Stopping your everyday activities can reduce your stress too.
- **To become aware of your body sensations.** Your body is like a barometer for your stress levels. To notice how your body feels will help you tune in to what's going on within you. For example, a pain in your neck can remind you to take a break from working on your computer before that turns into a migraine.
- **To notice your emotions.** Lack of awareness of your emotions can be a stressor in itself. If you're feeling angry, you can work out why. If you don't know you're feeling angry, it may just continue to build until you explode at whomever seems to be nearby.
- **To take a step back from whatever you're doing.** The mini-meditation is an opportunity to take a step back. You can then interpret things from this bigger picture. For example, if you're really stressed about an upcoming exam, the mini-meditation may remind you that you can only do your best. The exam is important, but doing badly isn't the end of the world.

The mindful pause has three steps. Allow about a minute for each step.

Step 1. Awareness of Body Sensations, Feelings, and Then Thoughts

Become aware of your body. Try to sit up straight if you're slouching. Gently open up your chest if your posture is closed. Hold your head up if you can. Notice what your body feels like, without judging yourself, as best you can. Which parts are tense? Which parts hurt? Which parts feel fine?

Then become aware of your feelings. How do you feel right now? You don't need to judge your feeling. Just notice the emotion and label it with a single word in your mind, like *sad*, *tired*, or *anxious*.

Next, turn your attention to your thoughts. Try imagining your mind as the sky and your thoughts like clouds. Place your thoughts on the clouds. Notice them come and go.

Step 2. Breath Awareness

Become conscious of the natural flow of your own breathing. Notice your breathing wherever you can—your nose, chest, or belly. See if you can totally accept your breathing just as it is.

Is your breathing shallow or deep? Is it smooth or not? How does the temperature of the air you breathe in differ from the air you breathe out?

Step 3. Connecting Your Awareness with Breath and Body

Now allow your attention to open up. Be aware of your whole body as you sit or stand here. Include your breathing, which of course is another sensation in your body. Get a sense of your whole body breathing if you can. Maybe play with feeling your breathing flowing up and down your body. Notice whether any tensions in your body stay the same or soften. Finish with holding a gentle smile on your face for a few seconds.

Consider how fortunate you are to have this time to practice a mindful pause for your own health and well-being. Congratulate yourself for having taken the time to pause.

TIP Just think *ABC* to remember the steps in the mindful pause. A stands for awareness of body, thoughts, and feelings; B stands for breath awareness; and C stands for connecting breath and body awareness together.

VARIATION: You can do this mindful pause while walking slowly or lying down.

GOING DEEPER: Begin by being clear about your intention for the practice. Set a timer for three times a day to practice the mindful pause. See if you can stop whatever you're doing to do the practice. And try doing the pause without an audio guide to see what effect that has. When practicing, see if you can keep your body absolutely still, including your eyes behind your eyelids. Keep your body relaxed yet upright and dignified in its posture. You can extend the practice for 10 minutes or longer if you have time.

Reflection

What did you notice about the mindful pause? What effect did the mindful pause have?

Discovering and Responding to Your Stress Signs

Angela worked for a furniture company. Her work was demanding, involving driving all over the country. It wasn't unusual for her to drive hundreds of miles each week, sometimes away from home for days at a time. The year she was burned out from stress, she'd driven more than 100,000 miles.

"I loved the buzz of the job," she said. "It was stressful, but I loved it." At first she just worked during the week, but as her responsibilities grew, she started working on weekends too.

Angela didn't have a social life, but that didn't seem to matter to her. Then she found a boyfriend. Making time for him on top of all the work proved to be really difficult. The pressure started to feel overwhelming. She started to feel lethargic all the time. Then, on a Monday morning, she just couldn't get out of bed. She could move her fingers and toes, but that was about it. She had no energy to move her arms and legs at all.

When she managed to get to the doctor, Angela was told that she was "burned out with stress." She found that hard to believe at first. Yes, life was stressful, but she enjoyed it for the most part. On further reflection, however, she discovered she didn't have a balance between work and the rest of her life.

Work had taken over her whole life. She'd been living habitually, automatically, without stopping to notice what was going on.

She spent a lot of time over the next few months at home, sleeping in bed. Gradually things started to improve. But when things did get better, she would push herself too much, like she did before, and ended up shattered, in bed for days.

Before she ended up seeing her doctor, there had been signs that Angela was under too much stress: a long-term lack of sleep, an unwillingness to socialize with friends and family, worrying thoughts going around and around in her head, and a constant feeling of being driven to work. Her body was completely tense. Unfortunately, she wasn't aware (mindful) enough to notice them—she just didn't know what to look for.

After joining a local mindfulness class and practicing the meditations for a number of months, she began to feel better. She began to be more sensitive to the needs of her body; she could actually notice her stress signs. The mindfulness revealed that when her stress rose there was a slight tightening in her throat. That was a signal for her to slow down and take a little mindful pause. Before, without mindfulness of her bodily sensations, she didn't even notice this sign, let alone the other tension all over her body. Angela felt meditation was for her one of the key factors in her path back to well-being.

You may see a commonality between this story of Angela's experience and what Anastasia experienced at the beginning of this chapter. They both were working hard with a lower level of awareness of their own emotions and bodily sensations. Without this awareness, the danger signs of excessive stress can't be seen.

Reflection

Take a few minutes to reflect on the last time you were under too much pressure and felt high levels of stress. Then answer the questions that follow, which may help give greater clarity about your stress.

1. What was the cause of your high level of stress?
2. What were the physical sensations that you felt when your stress levels rose? Where exactly in your body did you feel the sensations (e.g., tension, tightness, tingling, throbbing)?
3. How did you feel emotionally when your stress levels got too high (e.g., anxious, sad, frustrated, shy)?
4. What thoughts did you have when your stress levels got too high (e.g., "I can't cope"; "Why is he acting like this?")?

> 5. How do you react toward other people when your stress levels rise too much (e.g., ignore them, get angry, avoid them)?
> 6. What did you do when your stress levels became too high (e.g., took a break, worked harder, went to sleep, ate lots of chocolate, ignored it)?

As you go through this course, you'll continue to identify that your stress levels are beginning to get too high and learn ways to deal with rising stress levels. In this way, you can respond to your stress before it gets too high using mindfulness.

For example, consider Jay, who'd been struggling to get a new contract. He worked in the brand promotion business, and January was always a quiet time for him. After all the expenses of Christmas, money was tight. Living alone in London and not having enough money to heat his house felt increasingly frustrating. He woke up one Monday morning feeling extremely stressed. The stress kept rising as he thought about his situation and what could happen if he didn't manage to find any work over the next few weeks. Then he remembered what he'd learned in an MBSR class. He stopped and took a mindful pause. Rather than allowing the stress to rise higher, he caught the feeling early. He repeated this several times during the day, and with a

---

Research Corner: Mindfulness Could Help with Many Diseases by Reducing Inflammation

Many different diseases are associated with chronic inflammation in the body, including rheumatoid arthritis, psoriasis, inflammatory bowel disease, and asthma.

An exciting piece of research carried out in 2013 on about 60 people compared one half, who did an MBSR course like the one in this book, with the other half, who did a health enhancement program (HEP) that included walking, balance, agility, core strength, nutritional education, and music therapy. The study was carried out by Melissa A. Rosenkranz, PhD, and colleagues at the University of Wisconsin–Madison, and published in the journal *Brain, Behavior, and Immunity*.

Both groups were then stressed by being asked to give a 5-minute on-the-spot speech on a given topic and then challenged to 5 minutes of mental arithmetic. Both groups had a reduction in the stress hormone cortisol, but the group that trained in MBSR had a significantly lower inflammation response too. This suggests mindfulness could be an important approach to managing lots of diseases.

more centered, grounded state of mind, he called up some old contacts and managed to find work. As you can see, Jay was able to spot his stress signs and then use mindfulness to take control of it.

Breath as an Anchor for Your Experience

If your mind is chattering out of control, and your feelings are swirling around like a spicy soup on the boil, rest assured you're not alone. In a busy, modern 24/7 society, the constant stimulation, choices, and challenges whip up your thoughts and emotions. And when you're in this state of mind, you're much more likely to react automatically and unhelpfully to the stressors in your life.

One excellent way of managing your thoughts is to make use of your breathing. Using mindfulness of your breath to cope with stress can sound overly simplistic, but I'd urge you to try it before judging the approach. The calming effect occurs through use of your breath to anchor you in the present moment. And the more you use your breath to come to the present, the easier and more effective it becomes.

Take a moment to consider an anchor: the function of an anchor is to stop a ship from drifting aimlessly in the ocean. The anchor is always available on the ship, and wherever the ship goes, the anchor goes with it. Whenever the ship needs to stop, someone simply drops the anchor.

In the same way, wherever you go, your breath goes! Fortunately, you can't run away from your breathing, or leave your breathing at home when you go out for the day. Your breathing is with you, day and night. What you may forget is to actually pay attention to the feeling of your breathing from time to time. But whenever you want to stop, you can focus your attention on your breathing as an anchor to bring you into the here and now.

Breathing is a fascinating part of being human, one of those unique functions that can be both automatic and partially controlled. Your heartbeat is different, for example. Your heart is beating day and night, tirelessly. But you can't stop your heart beating for even a few seconds, as you can with your breathing. You can't instantly stop digestion or your immune system, either. Breathing is both automatic and under your control. There are very few other systems in the body that are so automated and yet under your control too.

Relaxation techniques often make use of deep breathing. This is because your breathing is intimately linked to the system in your body responsible for relaxation. Feelings of relaxation often occur when you breathe slowly and deeply. Mindfulness of breath is slightly different. In mindful breathing, you don't need to control the rate or depth of your breath. Instead, you simply turn your attention to your breathing just as it is, without judgment.

Tales of Wisdom:
The Meditator Who Aced His Final Exams

Here's a story I heard from a Buddhist monk. Before he became a monk, he was studying science at a top university in England. He had his final exams in the last year—and they were final! Everything that he'd learned in all the years at university was tested in six consecutive days. Each day he had a 3-hour exam in the morning and another 3-hour exam in the afternoon. It was grueling—a torture! Everyone kept telling him his whole future depended on the results of these exams, which didn't help. The pressure was seriously on. He had already learned meditation, and so he decided to have a big breakfast every morning and a nice dinner in the evening, but no lunch. Instead of lunch he went home and meditated for about half an hour. Every day when he did this, first the thoughts about the past exam came up. He let them go; no point thinking about that now. Then worries about the exam to come kept arising; he let them go. Worrying about it wouldn't help. And then he became aware of something incredible: as he became more present, he noticed his whole body was literally shaking with nervousness! His mind had been so full of thoughts, he hadn't noticed this at all. With a bit more meditation, his body began to settle down. He realized something amazing that day: it's possible for the body to be completely stressed and not to notice due to a barrage of thoughts. And a kind, caring, mindful awareness can relax and ease the body. Without this bodily awareness, stress can turn into something more serious, like an emotional burnout.

Needless to say he aced his exams. In fact, he was the only person who was smiling as he walked in to do the final exam on the final day; everyone else was completely mentally drained. So if you're facing a bunch of exams, try this approach!

PRACTICE: Mindfulness of Breath Meditation

 10 minutes.

This is the simplest and perhaps most powerful meditation practice of them all. By simple, I don't mean that being aware of your breathing is an easy thing to sustain. But the idea is very simple. Become aware of your breathing. When your mind wanders, bring your attention back.

That's it! No need to judge or criticize or anything else. Just awareness of breath. Try practicing this without a guided audio and see how you do.

1. Find a chair and sit up relatively straight, away from the back of the chair if you can. No need to be rigid or too uncomfortable. At the same time, avoid slouching. Adopt a dignified, yet comfortable posture. (See the drawing below.) Set a timer for about 10 minutes. Gently close your eyes if that feels okay with you.

> "I find mindful breathing deeply nourishing for my body and mind. It took a while to accept that my mind will wander, but now I love practicing mindfulness of breath— that's my favorite practice."

2. Take a deep, full breath. Feel the air filling your lungs and being released.
3. Allow your breathing to be natural now. Feel the sensation of your breathing around your nose, throat, chest, or down in your belly area; wherever is easy for you.
4. Keep your attention on the feeling of your breath as best you can.
5. Each time your mind wanders, notice what sort of thought you were having. And identify it as *planning*, or *worrying*, or *past*, or *ruminating*, or however you wish to label the thought stream. You could just use the label *thinking* if you prefer.
6. Then, without a need for criticism or self-judgment, gently guide

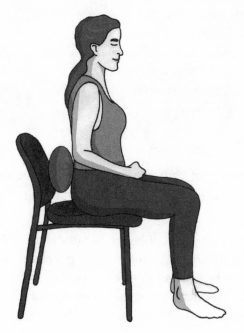

your attention once again to the sensation of your breathing. Be friendly with yourself when you bring your attention back rather than criticizing yourself.

7. When the timer sounds, slowly open your eyes if they've been closed.

VARIATION: You can also try the meditation while standing up or lying down to see what affect this has.

GOING DEEPER: Try to keep your body and eyes as still as possible while you do the meditation. If you normally do the practice with eyes closed, keep them open and softly gaze downward to see what effect that has. And if you normally have your eyes open, try closing them. Notice how each breath may be slightly different from the next one. Try feeling the breath with an attitude of affection and warmth, as if you're watching a baby or beautiful sunset or a loved one. And notice your intention for the practice before you start. Ask yourself, "What is my intention for practicing mindfulness?"

Reflection

What did you notice in your body, mind, and emotions in this practice?

The most common response people have is: "My mind was all over the place. I can't meditate." Remember, as I've mentioned before, a wandering mind is quite normal and natural. The aim of mindfulness is not to quiet the mind. The aim is to gently raise your level of awareness. So your wandering mind is a stepping-stone for you to notice the patterns with which your mind works.

> To *notice* that your mind was wandering really is a positive experience—it's a moment of mindfulness.

You may find mindfulness of breath a particularly challenging practice. Being mindful of your breathing may bring up feelings of anxiety, and perhaps your breathing starts to get more rapid or uncomfortable. If the exercise was not a pleasant experience, you may want to stop the practice or think you're doing the meditation wrong. That's totally understandable. But I would urge you to persevere with the technique. If you avoid the practice because you're trying to avoid feelings of anxiety, this may work in the short term, but in the long term you're avoiding your feelings, and this just makes the emotion more likely to return. If you can kindly and gently and curiously continue to move toward the uncomfortable feeling, your breathing is likely to settle and become a more comfortable and soothing experience.

(TIP) If you find your mind wanders continuously and you feel frustrated, you can try labeling each breath to give you a clearer focus. You can do this in three ways. Either you can say to yourself "in" or "in-breath" each time you breathe in, and "out" or "out-breath" each time you breathe out. Or you can say to yourself "breathing" each time you breathe in, and "smiling" as you breathe out. Or you can do this by saying "one" on the first in breath, "two" on the next out-breath, "three" on the next in-breath, and so on, until you get to 10. If you get to 10. Most likely, your mind will wander off to your shopping list or that argument you had with someone. When your mind comes back, begin again from 1.

Reflection:
Discoveries from Week 1 Mindfulness Experiments

Now's the time to reflect on how your mindfulness experiments have been going in the last week.

What did you discover in the week that's just passed? Did you do the mindful experiments? What's going well? What's not going well? Do you have a mindfulness buddy, and if so, are you in touch? What needs to change this week, if anything?

Note: This is not a chance to beat yourself up if you didn't do the meditations; it's a chance to explore what happened. What thoughts got in the way? How can you *encourage* yourself rather than just force or discipline yourself?

Mindfulness Meditation FAQs

Q: **I kept falling asleep in the body scan. Is that wrong?**

A: Nope! There's no right or wrong, no matter what happens. If you keep falling asleep in the body scan, try doing it at a different time of day and ensure you've had enough sleep. And try a different posture, like sitting or perhaps even briefly standing! Also notice what your mind is doing. Sometimes your mind makes you fall asleep to avoid the experience of the body scan. But don't worry if you keep falling asleep; the most important thing is to keep practicing.

Q: I felt anxious/more pain/depressed/worried—what do I do?

A: All sorts of different thoughts, feelings, and bodily sensations can come up as part of meditation. (Remember Anastasia's confusion when she found herself crying?) You can't control that. What you can control is how you respond to them. So bring a quality of curiosity and openness to these experiences and see what happens. No experience lasts forever, so watch the experience arise and pass away.

Q: I started to cry in my meditation. What's going on?

A: It's perfectly normal for tears to come up in meditation practice. Some teachers even go as far as to say you haven't ever experienced a deep meditation if you've never cried in a meditation. Sometimes, emotions that you haven't addressed in your past or hurts that haven't been processed come to the surface. It can bring tears to your eyes. And that's a very healthy experience. Be kind to yourself, try placing your hand on your heart, and keep going if you can. It will pass.

Q: I couldn't feel my feet/legs/anything. What's happening?

A: If you can't feel a sensation, that's perfectly okay. That's quite normal, especially at the beginning. The idea is to just notice the absence of sensation. If it's too frustrating for you, you could try slightly tensing or moving that body part to see if you can feel that sensation. But if you can, just accept the experience as it is. You may find yoga easier, as there are more sensations available when you're stretching your body.

Q: I found it boring. What can I do about that?

A: Boredom is a normal reaction to this practice. Even if you feel bored, keep going. Boredom is just an emotion, and it will pass. Try not to *react* to the emotion of boredom, but instead see if you notice where you feel it in your body, how powerful it is, and when it eventually passes. You can only "progress" in meditation when you can embrace the fact that boredom will come and go from time to time. Eventually you'll find your daily activities less boring, as well as your meditation.

Home Experiments: Week 2

Here are the daily mindfulness experiments for Week 2.

Body Scan

You are also invited to continue practicing the body scan meditation, whether you're doing the mini or full exercise. Continue to use the audio to guide you in the practice.

Pleasant Experience

This week you can experiment with recording one "pleasant experience" that you have on a daily basis. This doesn't have to be anything huge or life changing. Simply hearing a bird singing, someone holding a door open for you, enjoying the taste of your dinner, or someone smiling at you in a coffee shop is a pleasant experience. The key is to note down your thoughts, feelings, and body sensations at the time. For example, if the server smiled at you in a coffee shop, you may record: "Thought—'that's nice that she's smiling.' Feeling—'happy.' Body sensation—'smile on my own face, opening and warmth in my chest.'"

Mindful Pause

You're also invited to try the mindful pause three times a day. If you're doing the mini-course, you can do the mindful pause once a day. You'll probably find it easier if you decide when you'll do your mindful pauses. You can remember to do the practice by putting an alarm on your phone or setting an appointment with yourself in your journal.

Mindful Booster

This week's mindful booster is to brush your teeth with the opposite hand. If you are right-handed, use your left hand. And if you're left-handed, use your right hand. Simple!

You may be thinking, how is brushing with my left hand helping me with my stress?! Remember, by doing something different from your normal routine, you're becoming less automatic and more mindful. And greater mindfulness creates a greater awareness of not only the act of brushing your teeth but also your thought and emotional patterns, which may be currently wired to compound your stress.

Week 2

Day	Mini-Course	Full Course
1	Mini-body scan 1 × Mindful pause Mindful booster: brush your teeth with your other hand	Body Scan 1 × Mindfulness of breath meditation 3 × Mindful pause Write down a pleasant experience you had today. Record thoughts, feelings, and body sensations. Mindful booster: brush your teeth with your other hand
2	Mini-body scan 1 × Mindful pause Mindful booster: brush your teeth with your other hand	Body scan 1 × Mindfulness of breath meditation 3 × Mindful pause Write down a pleasant experience you had today. Record thoughts, feelings, and body sensations. Mindful booster: brush your teeth with your other hand
3	Mini-body scan 1 × Mindful pause Mindful booster: brush your teeth with your other hand	Body scan 1 × Mindfulness of breath meditation 3 × Mindful pause Write down a pleasant experience you had today. Record thoughts, feelings, and body sensations. Mindful booster: brush your teeth with your other hand
4	Mini-body scan 1 × Mindful pause Mindful booster: brush your teeth with your other hand	Body scan 1 × Mindfulness of breath meditation 3 × Mindful pause Write down a pleasant experience you had today. Record thoughts, feelings, and body sensations. Mindful booster: brush your teeth with your other hand

Day	Mini-Course	Full Course
5	Mini-body scan 1 × Mindful pause Mindful booster: brush your teeth with your other hand	Body scan 1 × Mindfulness of breath meditation 3 × Mindful pause Write down a pleasant experience you had today. Record thoughts, feelings, and body sensations. Mindful booster: brush your teeth with your other hand
6	Mini-body scan 1 × Mindful pause Mindful booster: brush your teeth with your other hand	Body scan 1 × Mindfulness of breath meditation 3 × Mindful pause Write down a pleasant experience you had today. Record thoughts, feelings, and body sensations. Mindful booster: brush your teeth with your other hand

SIX

Week 3

The Joy and Value of Living in the Present

> "What day is it?"
> "It's today," squeaked Piglet.
> "My favorite day," said Pooh.
> —A. A. MILNE

INTENTIONS

+ *To discover the true value of living in the present.*

+ *To explore mindfulness of breath meditation, the body scan, and mindful stretching approaches to bringing you into the here and now.*

+ *To uncover how to enjoy mindful walking.*

+ *To understand why your brain gets lost in stories and how to come back to the present moment.*

WHEN MIGUEL first learned meditation, about 10 years ago, he *thought* he was a focused person, living in the present. During the day he worked as a magazine editor, and in the evening he spent his time writing for various websites and other magazines. His mind was always on several things at the same time; he was a "multitasker."

He began to use mindfulness meditation to help with his sleep. He'd always been a bit of an insomniac, and he slotted a daily 10-minute mindfulness meditation into his busy schedule to see if it would help. He began to sleep longer and wake up more refreshed. The meditation was the only "downtime" that he had during his day. But he didn't apply mindful living to the rest of his life.

Miguel had an ongoing issue with his weight—it went up and down like a yo-yo. He was often on the latest fad diet, and exercise was like a military regimen for him. However, during his time at his last stressful job, Miguel had gained an extra 70 pounds, far more than he'd ever gained before. This shocked him. No matter how much effort and willpower he mustered, his weight just kept rising this time. He felt scared, confused, and frustrated.

Then one day, after one of his meditations, he thought, "What if I'm gaining this weight because I'm not really paying attention to what I'm doing?" This was a huge lightbulb moment for him! He began to watch himself very carefully and discovered he was absolutely right. Rarely did he actually taste his food, and everything was done in a rush. Practically all activities he engaged in involved multitasking. He had completely lost touch with his senses. He never looked up to see the clouds in the sky, feel the breeze against his skin, or take in his partner's smile. He had become disengaged with life, living a habitual, automatic, goal-driven, future-focused life. The incessant thinking in his brain sucked up all his attention.

He decided to be more present and to end an endless cycle of shame and self-criticism that he could now hear in his head. All the usual diet plans he'd tried seemed to use self-criticism to motivate the dieter, which was incredibly stressful. His meditation had taught him to live from one moment to the next, without judgment. He'd also noticed with his own dog that effective training is based on praising small, good behaviors rather than punishing undesirable behavior. So he decided to use the same approach in his own life, and to stop adopting the constant cycle of diet fads and punishments when he failed. He was going to be kind to himself and take small, positive steps to manage his weight, with mindfulness.

When Miguel meditated, his intention shifted to one based on self-kindness and respect. He deserved this time. And he balanced self-acceptance with a clear need to change his habits and behavior.

As he became more present with himself, he naturally also became more present with his food. His reactive, mindless eating began to dissolve, and the almost childlike joy of living in the present returned. He noticed that a lack of presence had meant there was no gap between the desire to eat something and actually eating that food. Now, when he saw a piece of cake, there was a space. Time for him to reflect and decide what to do. Time to take a mindful pause and make a choice. Time to be grateful that he had a meal available to him in the first place.

And most important, on the days he slipped up, Miguel didn't have to mentally punish himself. Instead, he remembered that self-compassion and presence are more important: not berating himself for an action that had already happened. He took a deep breath, came back to the present moment, and resolved to try again with a smile. He was awake to those moments of stress and took mindful action to reduce them.

Miguel's weight began to drop, pound by pound, week by week. He lost all the weight he had gained, this time at a healthy rate. Several years later his weight is still down, and he often shares the benefits of living in the present moment with anyone interested to listen.

The Value of Being Present

For Miguel, turning his attention to the present moment was critical to helping him manage his weight. He was then able to notice his eating habits and the overly self-critical commentary from his mind. He then took action, being kind to himself whether or not he was successful with his eating plan. It all started with being present in his own life.

As a human being, your brain is wired to think about the past and predict the future, as well as to connect with the present moment. But in our modern society, living in the present moment isn't really valued. It's easy to become a constant planner, forever thinking about your schedule for this week, this month, this year, and even this decade. But what about now? If you're constantly planning, you never arrive. This constant planning but lack of actually connecting with the moment is an easy mistake to make. If you're in this boat, you're certainly not alone.

Here's one of my favorite quotes, which I keep up on my noticeboard to remind me to live in the now:

> First, I was dying to finish my high school and start
> college. And then I was dying to finish college and start
> working. Then I was dying to marry and have children.
> And then I was dying for my children to grow old
> enough so I could go back to work. But then I was dying
> to retire. And now I am dying . . . And suddenly I realized
> . . . I forgot to live. Please don't let this happen to you.
> Appreciate your current situation and enjoy each day.
> —AUTHOR UNKNOWN

Sound familiar? I'm not advocating every second of your life be lived in the here and now; that's unrealistic and thinking in a perfectionistic way. But a better balance needs to be found. Researchers have discovered that people spend only about half of their time paying attention in the present moment and the other half in thoughts about the past and future. So, if you lived to age 80, you'd have spent 40 years of your waking life thinking about what happened yesterday or last month or planning and worrying about the future. That's a lot. It's more enjoyable and valuable to spend the precious few years you have on this planet actually living in the moment. I often joke that there's a new, free technique to double your lifespan: it's called mindfulness.

Mindfulness offers a set of practical tools, exercises, and attitudes to help you live in the present and make the present moment a more enjoyable and interesting place to be in. After all, the present moment is the only place where you can think, create, learn, grow, and take action.

Thought Is Not the Enemy

If you're thinking, that doesn't mean you're not mindful. If you are consciously choosing to think and reflect on what happened yesterday, and you know that you're thinking about yesterday, that's mindfulness. If you're consciously deciding to plan and choose what to do next month, and you know that you're doing so, that's mindfulness too. Mindful thinking is a conscious, deliberate observation of your thinking happening, without getting caught up in the thought process.

There is a time to deliberately think and plan and a time to connect with your senses. If you're at work, you probably need to spend a good deal of time thinking and taking action. But if you're walking along the beach, in a forest, or even walking home from work, that's the time to be present. To feel the gentle breeze against your skin, to notice the rose in a front yard, to hear a plane in the distance and the crunching of leaves under your feet.

> "Suddenly, the penny dropped. I don't need to battle with my thoughts. What a relief! I had always thought I was a failure at meditation because I couldn't shut my brain up. Now I focus on my breathing and let my mind carry on—and strangely, it seems to be quieter!"

Thoughts will always arise and pass away, just like the sun always rises and sets. You don't fight with the sunrise or sunset—you accept that that's the nature of the sun. In the same way, you don't need to fight your thoughts. It's the nature of thoughts to arise and pass away in your mind. In mindfulness, you learn to step back and watch the thoughts.

Even judgment and self-criticism can be mindful. If you are *aware* that your mind is judging, criticizing, or feeling anxious, then you're not lost in that feeling. That's what Miguel did in the earlier example: he saw how his mind was criticizing him. That's mindfulness. He then began to use a more

---

Research Corner:
A Wandering Mind Is an Unhappy Mind

A study by Matthew Killingsworth at Harvard University tracked the thoughts, feelings, and actions of 2,250 volunteers on their smartphones. They found people's minds wander 47% of the time. People reported that they are happiest when they are in the present, and higher levels of happiness are linked to lower levels of excessive stress. The study was aptly titled "A wandering mind is an unhappy mind." This seems to add further evidence for what many meditation practitioners in the East have been recommending: spend more time paying attention to whatever you're doing in the present moment rather than letting your mind go and wander wherever it pleases.

---

friendly approach to himself to help reduce his stress and increase his sense of well-being, giving him the strength to manage his weight.

By learning to live in the present, you're able to step back from your thoughts and see them as just that: thoughts. And your feelings of anxiety arising from stress can also be seen as an experience that arises and passes away, like all other emotions. By dissociating from the feeling, you're able to stop reacting and compounding the emotion.

The first time I learned the value of living in the present moment in an Eastern philosophy class, I was hooked! Before learning to be mindful, I was a constant thinker, and I wasn't aware of it. I was lost in thinking when I was driving, when I was walking, and when in conversation. I didn't think paying attention to my surroundings or my own bodily sensations was useful in any way. Why would I? I had never thought of cultivating that background quality that makes us all human but is so easily forgotten: awareness itself. My belief was life was short and shouldn't be wasted—and by spending all my time planning for the future, I'd have a better life, as would those around me. I didn't *value* present-moment living because I didn't know its importance.

All of life is experienced in the present moment. The here and now. There is no other place to live a fulfilling life. The past was in the present moment. The future will be in the present moment. So use mindfulness to make the moment a more fully experienced one, where you can make conscious decisions for both you and those you come in contact with.

Every experience you've ever had, every thought that's
popped into your mind, every trip, every success

and failure, all your hopes and dreams happen
in the present moment.

Dealing with Multitasking Stress

One of the main ways you may be missing out on present-moment living is through multitasking. Everyone multitasks, some more and some less. Modern technology encourages it. You may text while driving, watch TV while eating, and check your e-mail while speaking on the phone.

You probably multitask out of habit. The idea is you try to get more things done in less time. After a while, it becomes a powerful habit that's hard to break. My friend told me yesterday that he recently realized, after losing his job and starting a business that isn't taking off, that he's checking his e-mail and Twitter account about 20 times an hour! This is draining his energy and focus, and he knows it is making him more inefficient but is struggling to break the habit.

WHAT'S THE PROBLEM?

Rapidly switching attention from one thing to another actually diminishes your ability to do one thing at a time. So you have a greater chance of distracting yourself in the future with yet more multitasking.

WHAT'S THE SOLUTION?

If you're really addicted to multitasking, start small. Set aside a period of time where you will just focus on the task at hand. Make sure you turn off any possible distractions. As your ability to single-task increases, try longer periods of time. Each time your mind wanders, simply and kindly bring your attention back, just like in meditation. In this way, your life becomes a meditation!

When working on my computer, I set a timer on my phone for 30 minutes. I do one task during that time and then take a 5-minute break to have a mindful stretch, drink some water, and take a mental step back from my work. This has hugely improved my productivity, and I feel my stress is much lower. Stretching every half hour is better for my body, too. Try once every hour if every 30 minutes sounds impossible to you.

I use an online calendar and have set times to check my e-mail and phone. I need to check e-mail only once or twice a day, and that's what I do—your job may require more. I save my most productive time of the day to do the most important tasks (the morning for me) and check e-mail when I'm less creative and need a break from tasks that require a lot of thought (early afternoon).

> ### Reflection
>
> To help you decide how often you need to check your messages, practice the mindful pause (see Chapter 5) and then ask yourself the following question: "If I'm totally honest with myself, what is the minimum number of times I can check my messages in a day?"
>
> Allow yourself some time to reflect on the question before writing down your answer. If it's fewer times than you currently check, begin to implement this new habit by scheduling time to check. Your ability to be mindful and focused will improve as a result.

Here are a few more tips for using technology mindfully. They are all based around taking control by setting boundaries:

• **Switch off the alerts sent when you get a new e-mail or instant message.** You'll be distracted by the sound and will be tempted to stop your current task to meet someone else's need, which may not be important. If this is not possible due to the nature of your work, see if you can find a solution by discussing it with your manager. A study in 2012 by researchers at the University of California found that employees who had their e-mail switched off had a lower heart rate variability (and therefore lower stress) and increased the amount of single-tasking. This led to greater productivity and well-being.

• **Turn off your phone for chunks of the day.** If your phone is on all day, it's like you're on call all day. Anyone can distract you from your task

---

Research Corner:
Enhance Your Brain by Reducing Multitasking

At Stanford University, Clifford Nass carried out a study on multitasking on 262 college students. He expected that regular multitaskers would be better able to complete a multitasking experiment than others.

He found the opposite. Chronic multitaskers were terrible at multitasking! And more interestingly, even when they were given one task to do, they did it less effectively. So the moral is, practice mindfully doing one task at a time to maximize your efficiency and minimize your stress.

whenever they wish. Designate periods of the day to just focus on your task if you can.

• **Avoid taking your work back home.** If you're checking e-mail at home, you're at work. Find time to separate work from your home life. Checking your work messages will raise your stress levels. If you have to check messages at home, do so earlier rather than later in the evening to prevent the stress from affecting your sleep.

• **Turn off your phone when driving.** Research by transport authorities and others have found speaking on the phone while driving is as dangerous as driving while drunk. And having a hands-free phone is not safer. Driving mindfully can and does save lives.

Bodily Sensations: A Powerful Way to Be Present

Your mind can pay attention fully to only one thing at any time, so one of the easiest ways to be in the present is to become aware of your bodily sensations. This is because your body is always in the present. If you're fully paying attention to your bodily sensations, you're not lost in thinking about what happened in the past or worrying about the future. You can't be both lost in thoughts and fully paying attention to your bodily sensations.

What do I mean by bodily sensations? Here are some examples:

- Aches
- Heat or cold
- Itching, tingling, or throbbing
- Lightness or heaviness
- Numbness
- Pressure
- Sharp or dull pain
- Tension or tightness
- An absence of sensation altogether

These sensations may not sound like a very exciting place to keep your attention. But once you focus your attention on bodily sensations, you discover a range of interesting aspects.

• You experience and notice that **bodily sensations are always changing**—they are temporary. They never stay exactly the same. They tend to rise and pass away, just as a wave gradually rises and falls. And if you seem to have a permanent sensation of pain, for example, even then the pain disappears when you fall asleep and there are moments in the day when the pain diminishes. Many people with chronic pain find mindfulness helps them notice times in the day when the pain is diminished or completely absent.

• **Feeling bodily sensations can be a pleasant experience.** People often describe the process as grounding or nourishing. Some people say tuning in to bodily sensations gives them a feeling of wholeness or completeness. There is pleasure to be discovered in simply being mindful of your bodily sensations at any time during the day.

• **Bodily sensations can accurately signal your current levels of stress.** You discover your bodily sensations are intimately linked to your emotional state. Pretty much all emotions have a component linked to sensation in your body. The body sensations that are linked to emotions are slightly different for different people. For you, anxiety may involve a tingling in the stomach and tightness in the shoulders, sadness may be a tightening in the chest and weakness in the muscles, happiness may involve a sense of opening in the chest area and a smile on the face and a sense of relaxation in your forehead. Stress may make you feel anxious or sad or angry, and you'll be able to sense these emotions in your body if you're mindful. You can then decide what you need to best take care of yourself.

• You find that **mindfulness seems to have a long-term positive effect on bodily sensations.** For example, when you feel tension in your body with

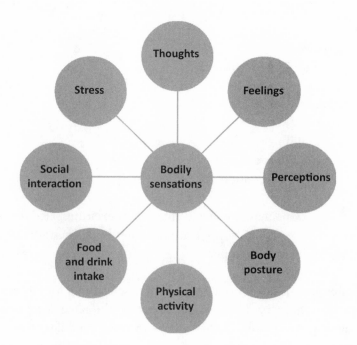

a kindly, curious, open, nonjudgmental awareness, the tension tends to ease. And if it doesn't, you are more accepting of the tension and so it's not so much a problem. Emotions also seem to process more effectively with mindful awareness. By noticing the dimension of bodily sensations when you're experiencing a difficult emotion, you're less likely to get lost in the "story" of the emotion and instead can allow the e-*motion* to do just that—keep moving!

• **You actually experience how thoughts affect your bodily sensations, for better or worse.** As emotions are linked to your thoughts, your thoughts affect your bodily sensations. When your attention dwells on stressful thoughts such as all the things on your to-do list, you're more likely to feel anxiety rising and have the bodily sensations that typically come with it. And even when you're not meditating but going about your everyday activities, whatever your senses take in is judged by your thoughts, and this affects your emotions and then bodily sensations. Just consider what effect the flavor of your favorite food has on your body. Or the smell of something unpleasant. Or the sight of a beautiful sunrise over a lake.

The truth is, many different factors affect your bodily sensation at any one moment, as can be seen in the diagram on the facing page. You can see how being aware of exactly how your body feels gives you a "report" of how things are going for you. So now you know why mindfulness often emphasizes awareness of your bodily sensations and how useful this can be in your everyday life, giving you information about how you're feeling and so helping you decide what you need to do to take care of yourself and reduce your stress.

> "After doing the body scan for a couple of weeks, I was walking down the stairs and actually felt my legs. I know it sounds crazy, but normally I don't feel them unless I'm hurt. Instead I was feeling my body and for the first time in literally years it felt good to just be alive and feel my body."

For example, I just practiced a mindful pause. Before the pause I had a feeling of a little headache and a need to get my work done. After doing the pause and tuning in to my bodily sensations, I noticed that the back of my neck was tense—and it released itself as I felt it along with a deep breath. I then noticed that my thoughts were going to a mini-workshop that I'm teaching this afternoon and haven't had time to plan yet. That little bit of stress was causing anxiety and probably my headache; the headache was not due to a lack of water or fresh air. So now I shall get on with planning that session, which I'm sure will lower my level of stress. This is a small example of a mindful way through stress.

Tales of Wisdom: The Three Questions

Once upon a time, an interesting thought came to a king. He thought if he could answer three questions, he wouldn't fail at anything he did. The questions were:

- When is the best time to do each thing?
- Who are the most important people to work with?
- What is the most important thing to do?

So he decided to consult a hermit, widely renowned for his wisdom. The king walked through a forest to find the hermit. The hermit was digging. The king asked the hermit his questions, but the hermit just kept digging. The king noticed the hermit was old and tired, so he offered his help. The king kept digging, until evening came. Tired, he stopped and asked the hermit for his advice again. The hermit said "Look, there's someone running—see who it is!"

A man came running through the woods and collapsed. He was bleeding around his stomach. The king rushed to look after him, washing and bandaging his wound, looking after him for hours. He then carried him to the hermit's hut, as the sun had set and it was getting cold. By this time the king was so exhausted that he fell asleep next to the wounded man.

The next morning, the king woke up and found the wounded man awake and smiling at him. "Forgive me!" said the man. "I was planning to kill you in revenge. I'm your enemy because you executed my brother. I was wounded by one of your bodyguards when I tried to enter the forest. But without your kindness last night, I would have surely died. Forgive me. I'm no longer your enemy. I'm your humble servant!"

The king was pleased to hear an enemy had turned into an ally.

The king still didn't have the answers to his questions. So he begged the hermit one more time to answer his three questions.

The hermit said: "You already have your answers. By being mindful of my needs in the present moment and helping, you met the wounded man. Being kind to him turned a potential killer into a friend."

1. The most important time is now. The present is the only time over which we have power.
2. The most important person is whomever you are with.
3. The most important thing is to do good to the person you are with.

And I'd like to add, if you happen to be on your own at any time, *you're* the most important person you're with, and the most important thing to do is to do good to *yourself*!

PRACTICE: Mindful Yoga

🕐 *10 minutes.*

🕐 *30 minutes.*

Audio tracks 9 (mini) and 10 (full).

At this point in your reading, consider practicing some mindful stretching and yoga. See Chapter 13 for an introduction to yoga and then carry out the mini or full yoga sequence, depending on which course you've chosen to do or which sequence you have time for right now. Alternatively, you can try out one of the sequences after reading the whole chapter (if you try both mini and full sequences, you can figure out which you want to try for the week's practices). You can also use the audio download to guide you in the practice. That's the easiest way for most people.

PRACTICE: Mindfulness of Breath Meditation

🕐 *10 minutes.*

🕐 *10 minutes.*

Audio track 12.

Let's now finish the yoga practice with mindfulness of breath meditation, ideally in an upright sitting posture. Sitting upright makes staying awake and in the moment a little easier. Traditionally the stretches in yoga were designed to help relax the body so that you could then practice meditation in a sitting posture comfortably. If you have time and space, practice some yoga stretches before engaging in this meditation. This meditation fits into either the mini or the full course, although it takes only 10 minutes. The instructions for the meditation are in Week 2.

Whenever you feel your bodily sensations, you're taking a step into the present moment. In this short sitting meditation, you can practice feeling your body sensations for 10 minutes.

Discovering Modes of Mind:
Doing and Being Mode

Chronic stress can generate difficult emotions like anxiety and sadness. When these emotions are fleeting, they are not a problem. But if the emotions stay with you for long periods, with high levels of intensity, you can find getting on with your daily activity more challenging. How can you let these emotions go?

To answer this question, you need to understand two different modes of mind, studied by researchers over the last 10 years: doing and being mode.

Doing mode is an important everyday mode of mind. Doing mode involves setting goals in your mind and taking action to achieve those goals. Working actively to finish the tasks on your to-do list is a classic example of doing mode.

Being mode is not about goals or change, but about allowing and accepting your present-moment reality. Being mode involves a connection with your senses. If you're fully in being mode, you don't get any of your tasks done. Watching a sunset with your attention fully focused, even for a few moments, is an example of pure being mode.

Some activities in life require more doing mode, and others require more being mode. Mindfulness offers you the ability to see whether you're in doing mode, being mode, or somewhere in between. You are then able to switch from one mode of mind to another. The diagram below shows how you can shift between using doing mode to achieve goals and using being mode to manage emotions. In this way, you are better able to handle the emotions that can arise from stress.

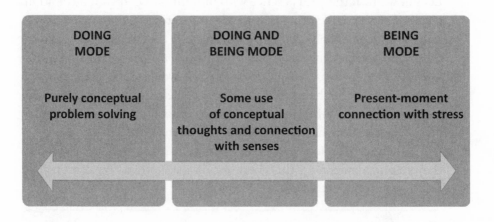

Don't think of doing as bad and being as good. *They both have to be balanced for a full and satisfying life.*

Let's take an example.

STUCK IN DOING MODE

You think, "My child is misbehaving, yet again." You feel anxious. You think, "What can I do? What if she behaves badly for the next 10 years? How can I cope with that?" You get angry with your child, really trying to make her stop kicking the sofa. She starts crying. You grab her, tell her not to misbehave, and get into a fight. You keep trying to think of action you can take to banish your anxiety.

MOVING BETWEEN BEING AND DOING MODE

You feel anxiety about your relationship with your husband. Rather than ignoring the feeling or trying to fix anything, you notice the sensation in your belly. You feel the tingling. You hear thoughts in your head but watch them like clouds passing through the sky, not engaging with them. You take a deep breath. You notice the sound of the tree in the breeze in your garden and a plane flying in the distance. Your shoulders start to relax, which makes you smile. The anxiety naturally lessens. You are living in the present with being mode.

You then engage doing mode and start thinking about how you can make things better between you and your husband tonight by treating yourselves to your favorite restaurant.

Doing mode is for getting things done. Being mode is for resting and dealing with emotions.

There is no such thing as a "bad" emotion. Emotions are just emotions. You're a human being, and human beings naturally have emotions. And emotions are not all pleasant—it's unrealistic to feel happy and stress-free *all* the time. You can cultivate a mind that is less likely to feel stressed, but this comes through learning and accepting all emotions that can come and visit you.

Emotions are not problems to be solved.
They are experiences to be felt.

Once you stop seeing emotions as all bad, you're less judgmental and self-critical. The emotions no longer need to be fixed. And so thoughts like "Why am I feeling so anxious? What's wrong with me?" don't come up so much. And if they do, you don't take those thoughts so seriously. You live in the present moment with your feeling, accept the emotion for what it is, and move on.

So another benefit of living in the present is a greater ability to process difficult emotions so they don't get stuck to you so much.

WALKING MINDFULLY: A WAY INTO BEING MODE

I love teaching mindful walking in my classes, especially to people who have never tried mindful walking before. Most people either find it funny or gasp with amazement at how little they knew about their own process of walking.

Normally you walk for a reason: you want to get somewhere. You walk to get a glass of water from downstairs or to pick up the milk from your local store. And so your attention is rarely on the process of walking itself; your focus is on the destination.

Mindful walking is different. When you practice mindful walking, your attention is in the present moment, not on what you're trying to do. Here are the aspects of the present moment that you could notice when doing mindful walking:

- Your breathing
- The sensations in your feet
- The sensations in your legs
- The air against your skin
- The sounds you hear
- The colors that you see
- The smells

"I felt really silly when I first tried mindful walking in the session. But once I actually gave my full attention to the process of walking and not my worries, it was freeing—it was like I was walking on the moon! I managed to give full attention to the moment and totally forgot about my work worries!"

Have you ever watched a young child walking? She is walking mindfully, fully connected with her senses. She sees the puddle and marvels at the color and usually jumps in! She's curious, enchanted, and not at all worried about how late she is. If she spots a beautiful flower, she will pluck it. If she hears a plane, she'll gaze and smile and say, "Wow." Imagine living like that? Well, you probably did live in that way as a child, at least some of the time, and so you do know how to live that way. Mindfulness is about rekindling that enthusiasm for the here and now. Exciting, isn't it?

PRACTICE: Mindful Walking

 5 minutes.

10 minutes.

Audio track 11.

This practice takes 5–10 minutes. As a beginner of mindful walking, I recommend you walk very slowly, somewhere you'll feel comfortable and safe. Most people start in their own homes or perhaps their yard. Here's how to do mindful walking:

1. **Set your intention.** Begin by being clear that for the next 5 minutes or so you're going to give your full attention to mindful walking. Ensure any potential distractions are reduced.

2. **Take three deep, mindful breaths.** This little ritual helps to send a signal to your brain that you're engaging in the mindful exercise now. The deep breaths also help to reduce the stress response in your body.

3. **Stand upright.** To begin with, you simply need to stand upright, and if you can balance, close your eyes for a few moments. Notice whether your body is tense or relaxed. Feel the distribution of weight on your feet and sway to the left and right, front and back, to find a central, balanced point so your weight is evenly spread between your feet.

4. **Lift, move, place.** As you walk, the process is made of three steps: lifting a foot, moving it in front of the other foot, and placing the foot. Then the process of lifting, moving, and placing switches to the other foot. So notice this cycle of lifting, moving, and placing. You can even say to yourself, "lifting, moving, placing" as you do so.

5. **Stop when your mind wanders.** As with any other meditation, your mind wanders—that's part of the experience. When you notice that your mind is lost in thoughts, stop walking, take three deep, mindful breaths, and then restart the process.

6. **Stop and turn around.** Once you reach the end of your room or yard, stop. Take a few moments to notice how you feel emotionally, as well as how your body feels physically. Then turn around slowly. Experience the process of turning around. Notice all the

different muscles involved and how you twist your body around. Then pause for a few moments before beginning your walk back.

7. **End the practice.** You can bring this gentle practice to an end with three mindful deep breaths again. Then see if you can be mindful with whatever you need to do next but giving the task your full attention. This is an example of a mindful transition from one activity to another.

(TIPS) Start with a slow speed, but remember, mindful does not equal slow. You can even practice mindfulness when sprinting!

If you walk in a circle, you don't need to stop and turn around when practicing at home or in a park or yard.

When you go for a normal walk in your everyday life, just give attention to one aspect of the experience. This could be your feet, your breathing, or the beauty of your surroundings. Whatever you like! There are no rules to mindful walking, as long as your intention is to be in the present moment and experience whatever happens unfold.

You can use this as a mindful booster whenever you like.

GOING DEEPER: See if you can go even slower. Take twice as long to take each step and see what else you can notice. Perhaps you'll observe how the rate of your breathing changes or discover new muscles that are involved when walking, such as your back muscles. Also, experiment with adding a little smile on your face to see what affect that has.

Walking Meditation FAQs

Q: I lose my balance when walking. What can I do?

A: Keep your eyes open, first of all! Some people mistakenly think they need to keep their eyes closed, but this isn't necessary. If you lose your balance because you're walking slowly, this is *very* common. Try walking near a wall when doing slow mindful walking so you don't fall over—that's important. You will get better at it once you have more practice; your brain is relearning to walk at a slower pace.

Q: I get overwhelmed by all the things I can notice and see. Help!

A: Many people have this issue when they walk outside, as there's so much to see! Try focusing on something simple, like the sensations of your feet on the ground. When your attention is drawn to your other senses, just softly bring your awareness back to the soles of your feet as you walk.

Q: Can I do mindful walking when walking briskly to work?

A: Yes! You can't notice the finer details of your bodily sensations when you walk quickly, but that's okay. See if you can stay in the moment instead of worrying about what's going to happen once you get to work. Or if you have a lot to think about, give yourself 10 minutes to think about the issues, but then make your intention to live in the moment and walk with mindfulness.

Q: Is mindful walking the same as walking meditation?

A: Yes, they are different terms for the same thing.

Q: I don't have time for mindful walking, as I'm so busy. What can I do?

A: Mindful walking doesn't take up any extra time. Whenever you walk, simply walk with mindful awareness of your moment-to-moment experience rather than constantly planning or worrying. There's a time to plan and a time to be mindful.

Q: Most of my day is spent at the office. How could I do some mindful walking there without looking stupid?

A: Just walk as you normally do and give your attention to the moment. Nobody will know that you're walking mindfully. That's undercover mindfulness!

Q: Is mindful walking really as good as normal meditation?

A: Yes. Meditation doesn't mean you need to be still. In the Buddhist tradition, for example, they consider four "postures" in meditation: sitting, lying down, standing, and walking. In retreats and workshops, often plenty of time is given to walking meditation.

Is Your Brain Lost in a Stressful Story?

You now know that one key aspect of stress is the thoughts that you believe to be true, that pop into your head. If your thoughts suggest all is well and you're in control, your stress levels stay balanced. However, if your thoughts dwell on the negative and make you feel out of control, your stress levels rise.

Thoughts usually come in the form of stories in your head. The human brain loves stories. Since ancient times, stories have been passed on from generation to generation. Literature is filled with stories, from Aesop's fables to the plays of Shakespeare. Historians often conjure up images of ancient cultures sitting around a fire telling each other stories.

Consider the brain a story-telling machine. From the moment you wake up in the morning, you're telling yourself the story of your own life. In the initial second or so of waking up, you're just present, without your story. Perhaps you've noticed this? And then your personal story comes rushing into awareness, usually without your awareness. Your brain reminds you who you are, where you live, and what you need to do. This is all an automatic process.

You're telling yourself stories about all sorts of people, situations, events, and challenges all the time. By becoming aware that you're telling yourself a story about a particular stressful situation, you can consider whether that story is actually true. By definition, being a story, it may not be totally true. Everyone sees stories differently.

Your sense of self is constructed in two ways: either using stories created over time, or through your present-moment experiences. If I asked, "Who are you?" you'd probably tell me your name. If I asked again, you would start telling me your story—where you were born, what you do for work, what you do in your spare time, and so on. But you can also *sense* who you are without your story. And you do this by connecting with your senses. That's where mindfulness comes in.

The story-telling brain, activating the default network, includes activity in the part of your brain responsible for memory. Waiting in a line at the local mall, your mind wanders, daydreams, and worries. But this network can also easily engage when you're taking a stroll through your local park. Rather than seeing the beauty, you can become caught up in your little world of concerns and worries. It is the story you tell yourself about your own life, the lives of other people you know, and how you all interact with each other.

There's nothing wrong with the narrative-based part of your brain. But you don't want to limit your life to your personal narrative, as it's easy to get lost in negative thoughts and emotions if you're not mindful. Evidence is mounting that the more you are continually lost in stories in your mind, the more susceptible you are to excessive stress and anxiety.

Fascinating research in 2007 by Norman Farb and colleagues at the University of Toronto tested one group that had completed an 8-week course in mindfulness meditation and a novice group that hadn't. The researchers discovered another network in the brain that activates when you connect with your senses—direct experience. This involves parts of the brain responsible for bodily sensations and for switching attention. This direct experience activation is a mindful state. You're living in the present moment—it is *being mode* in operation. As you walk through the park you notice the scent of the trees, the color of the flowers, and the sensations in your body.

The researchers found the mindfulness course group was more aware when they were lost in a narrative. The neural activity for the story-telling brain and the direct experience in their brains were more distinctly separated in the new meditators. They could therefore switch from the story-telling brain to a present-moment focus more easily.

You can't have both the narrative and direct-experience networks of your brain activated at the same time. So as you're strolling through the park, if you're lost in your default narrative network, you're more likely to dwell on your stressors. But there's good news. As soon as you begin to activate the direct-experience network part of your brain—which can be as simple as feeling your breath or the gentle breeze against your face—your narrative network calms down and the direct-experience network in your brain activates. You notice an old friend you've been meaning to talk to, a new path back home from the woods, and your stress levels begin to ease.

Reflection

Enter your answers in your journal if you like.

1. Try completing the following sentences to discover what the story-telling brain is telling you about yourself right now. Just note the first word or sentence that comes to mind; no need to think too much about it.

    I am . . .

    I am also . . .

    I live in . . .

    Today I need to . . .

    My childhood was . . .

    I'm grateful for . . .

    Life is . . .

The world is . . .

In the future I will . . .

I like myself because . . .

Other people are . . .

The purpose of life is . . .

I will be mindful by . . .

My stress is caused by . . .

I will reduce my stress by . . .

Here is an important question to consider: **Do you think your answers would change if you were in a really happy mood right now?** If so, are the answers absolute facts or just your current story?

2. Consider something that's causing you stress at the moment. What is the story you're telling yourself about the situation?

Now practice the Mindful Pause from Week 2 for a few minutes.

3. Now think about the wisest person you know. It may be someone you know personally and have respect for like your grandmother, an uncle, or a colleague at work. Or it could be someone you admire, like the Dalai Lama, Socrates, Gandhi, Martin Luther King, Jr., or Nelson Mandela.

    How would that person see this story if he or she were in your shoes?

    What action would this person take to overcome the challenge?

Now practice the Mindful Pause for a few minutes again.

Recalling your stressor, does it still cause as much stress? Do you have any ideas or solutions to help reduce the stress, even just a tiny bit?

INVICTUS

This is a poem that famously inspired the late Nelson Mandela during his decades of incarceration in South Africa. He used to read the poem to lift the spirits of fellow prisoners.

Out of the night that covers me,
Black as the Pit from pole to pole,
I thank whatever gods may be
For my unconquerable soul.
In the fell clutch of circumstance
I have not winced nor cried aloud.
Under the bludgeonings of chance
My head is bloody, but unbowed.
Beyond this place of wrath and tears
Looms but the Horror of the shade,
And yet the menace of the years
Finds, and shall find, me unafraid.
It matters not how strait the gate,
How charged with punishments the scroll.
I am the master of my fate:
I am the captain of my soul.
—WILLIAM ERNEST HENLEY (1875)

Reflection

What effect did this poem have on you? Write your thoughts in your journal if you like.

Reflection:
Discoveries from Week 2 Home Experiments

Here's an opportunity for you to reflect on how your meditation practice and experiments have been going over the last week. Consider each one in turn and make good use of your journal to reflect on how things have gone for you.

Body scan: You've been practicing the body scan for a couple of weeks now. Some people start to feel really bored with the practice; other people start to enjoy it. Neither is right or wrong. What has your experience been like in the last week?

Mindful pause: Did you remember to practice the mindful pause? If not, what can you do this week to remind yourself? If you did remember, what effect did the mindful pause have? For many of my students, the mindful pause is their most valuable practice.

Pleasant events calendar: Did you have a go at filling in this calendar? If not, can you schedule time to complete it this week? What patterns did you notice? You'll get a chance to explore the calendar in greater detail in a week's time.

Mindful booster: What did you discover when brushing your teeth with your other hand? Did the process make you feel more present and conscious rather than automatic? Some people find the process fascinating, whereas others get frustrated or just give up. What happened to you?

Home Experiments: Week 3

The recommended home experiments for you alternate this week. One day it's the body scan and the other day it's mindful yoga.

Body Scan

As you're alternating between the body scan and mindful yoga every day, notice what effect this is having on your practice. Around Week 3, I often find people getting particularly frustrated with the meditation as the novelty has worn off. So don't be surprised if you experience this with the body scan, and I warmly encourage you to persevere, despite what your mind is telling you!

Mindful Yoga

For the yoga, you can also either do 10 minutes or the full 30 minutes. If you're doing 10 minutes, try the exercises outlined in the mini-yoga sequence in Chapter 13. If you're doing 30 minutes, use both tracks from the yoga audio download—the mini followed by the full. Remember to do the exercises slowly and with kindly attention to your body and pay special attention to your breathing. Set a timer so you know when you've practiced for long enough or stop if you feel your body needs to stop.

Unpleasant Experience

As you recorded your pleasant experiences last week, this week you can try recording unpleasant experiences! Keep an attitude of curiosity and openness when you do this and remember to record your body sensations, thoughts, and emotions around the unpleasant experience. This may begin to reveal personal patterns that you haven't noticed before.

Mindful Booster

This week's booster is based on your daily walk. If you walk on the same route every day, try taking a different path this week. This may involve walking a little farther, or maybe just walking on the other side of the road. If you can't do that, just try walking in a really mindful way. Simply feel the sensations of your feet as you walk. Give attention to the soles of your feet, just as you focused on your breathing in the mindfulness of breath meditation—with curiosity, care, and patience.

(TIP) Walk a tiny bit slower than you normally do, to help get you out of your habitual way of moving and make you more conscious of your actions.

Mindful Pause

Continue to do the three mindful pauses every day. Or just once a day if that's all you can manage. That's great practice, and you'll be learning how to use the Mindful Pause to catch stress and meet it mindfully before it rises up too much.

Week 3

Day	Mini-Course	Full Course
1	Mini-yoga practice Note an unpleasant experience you had today and record thoughts, feelings, and body sensations. Mindful booster: take a different route home or simply walk mindfully	Full yoga practice 1 × Mindfulness of Breath Meditation 3 × Mindful Pause Note an unpleasant experience you had today and record thoughts, feelings, and body sensations. Mindful booster: take a different route home or simply walk mindfully

Day	Mini-Course	Full Course
2	Mini-body scan Note an unpleasant experience you had today and record thoughts, feelings, and body sensations. Mindful booster: take a different route home or simply walk mindfully	Full body scan 1 × Mindfulness of Breath Meditation 3 × Mindful Pause Note an unpleasant experience you had today and record thoughts, feelings, and body sensations. Mindful booster: take a different route home or simply walk mindfully
3	Mini-yoga practice Note an unpleasant experience you had today and record thoughts, feelings, and body sensations. Mindful booster: take a different route home or simply walk mindfully	Full yoga practice 1 × Mindfulness of Breath Meditation 3 × Mindful Pause Note an unpleasant experience you had today and record thoughts, feelings, and body sensations. Mindful booster: take a different route home or simply walk mindfully
4	Mini-body scan Note down an unpleasant experience you had today and record thoughts, feelings, and body sensations. Mindful booster: take a different route home or simply walk mindfully	Full body scan 1 × Mindfulness of Breath Meditation 3 × Mindful Pause Note down an unpleasant experience you had today and record thoughts, feelings, and body sensations. Mindful booster: take a different route home or simply walk mindfully
5	Mini-yoga practice Note an unpleasant experience you had today and record thoughts, feelings, and body sensations. Mindful booster: take a different route home or simply walk mindfully	Full yoga practice 1 × Mindfulness of Breath Meditation 3 × Mindful Pause Note an unpleasant experience you had today and record thoughts, feelings, and body sensations. Mindful booster: take a different route home or simply walk mindfully

Day	Mini-Course	Full Course
6	Mini-body scan Note an unpleasant experience you had today and record thoughts, feelings, and body sensations. Mindful booster: take a different route home or simply walk mindfully	Full body scan 1 × Mindfulness of Breath Meditation 3 × Mindful Pause Note an unpleasant experience you had today and record thoughts, feelings, and body sensations. Mindful booster: take a different route home or simply walk mindfully

SEVEN

Week 4

Understanding and Managing Stress

It's not stress that kills us, it is our reaction to it.
—HANS SELYE

INTENTIONS

+ *To discover the physiology of stress.*

+ *To find out how mindfulness helps you deal with stress.*

+ *To explore how to maintain peace in the face of pleasant and unpleasant experiences.*

+ *To practice some new mindful yoga sequences.*

SOFIA HAD suffered with anxiety since high school, and now, in her mid-twenties, she felt like she was reaching the breaking point. She wasn't sure how much more negativity her brain could take. She was always scared of spending time with other people, thinking how they were probably judging her for looking stupid and constantly frightened of saying the wrong thing. She was exhausted by the relentless fear of socializing with others that held a firm grip on her mind and body.

She'd tried some counseling, read countless books on reducing anxiety, and out of desperation decided to give meditation a try, having read about the benefits on an Internet forum. She didn't like the idea of meditation at all, first because it sounded religious and spiritual and she didn't believe in that stuff, and second because she had lost all hope of being able to help herself.

She got a mindfulness meditation CD and began to listen to the guidance for doing mindfulness of breath meditation. Through the exercise, she began to realize that by feeling her breath she could allow her negative thoughts about herself and others to dissolve gradually. Yes, her mind did keep coming back to her worries, but as the mindfulness audio advised, she repeatedly returned her attention to her breath. The more she practiced the more her anxiety diminished, as her awareness was more focused on breathing than her ruminating, self-defeating thoughts. She realized that these worries about what other people were thinking were just stories in her mind—they weren't necessarily true at all. She was just feeling anxious about false ideas her own mind had made up.

Sofia was hooked. She committed to practicing meditation every morning. The peace of mind she accessed through mindful breathing prevented her mind from getting into its habitual negative cycles at the start of the day. With that positive start, she felt less stress during the day and was more focused and present for the tasks she had to do.

Sofia's key discovery was that the human mind can fabricate stories that seem so real and frightening and yet actually are completely untrue. The wild mind can come up with hopeless ideas, and the low mood they generate creates a cycle of despair. She found that once you start to cultivate a greater level of self-awareness, you begin to naturally access those deep resources of inner serenity—a wellspring of hope.

Discover: The Physiology of Stress

In Chapter 1 you learned a little about the difference between pressure and stress. Medium levels of pressure can be energizing and motivating. But as the pressure rises to higher levels, as for Sofia, your body fully engages the stress response. What exactly is the stress response, and what happens in your body when the stress response is triggered? You'll find out in this section. If you feel stress is something that you experience more than others, I hope the following information will show you how universal the effects of stress are, and how understanding them can help us all reduce stress.

This doesn't mean all experts see stress in the same way. But, in fact, understanding stress from different perspectives can help you form a more complete picture of what stress is, its underlying causes, and the best ways of responding mindfully rather than reacting automatically. See which ideas resonate with you.

I've had a personal fascination with the subject of stress from a young age. When I first experienced a significant amount of stress, in college, I began to read about the subject. What I found most interesting was that stress is not just a casual word but a highly complex biological mechanism that has evolved over millions of years as a mode of living.

There are two key ways of looking at stress:

1. As the short-term **fight-or-flight response.**
2. According to the long-term effects of stress—**general adaptation syndrome.**

FIGHT OR FLIGHT

The stress response is often called the fight-or-flight response—the automatic, primitive reaction that prepares your body to attack or run away from a perceived threat to your survival. (Sometimes it's called the fight, flight, or freeze response because it can also make you freeze.) As described in Week 3, this mechanism has evolved over millions of years to protect you from harm and increase your chances of survival, with one result being an innate negativity bias among today's humans.

When you experience an external threat or just internal worries and concerns, the part of the brain called the hypothalamus is activated, which initiates a series of nerve cell firings as well as releasing chemicals like cortisol, adrenaline, and noradrenaline into your bloodstream. This combination of nerve cell activation and chemical release causes many changes. Your breathing rate and blood pressure increase, energy is directed away from your digestive and immune system and toward your muscles, and your reflexes quicken. Mentally, the more wise, intelligent, and rational part of your brain is shut down.

Essentially, this mechanism puts you into attack mode both physically and mentally to prepare you for the threat. If you were a prehistoric human and spotted a tiger, the fight-or-flight response could make the difference between life and death. Then and now, the surge of stress hormones gives you the strength to run away or fight an aggressor, to lift a car off your loved one, or to escape a burning building.

When you are in fight-or-flight mode, your brain scans the environment and perceives everything in your surroundings as a threat to survival. As if a thief has entered your home, you perceive every moment or sound as a sign of danger—even if it's just the wind blowing the curtains. A harmless comment is seen as an attack. You overreact to feedback. Your thoughts are irrational. Your fear becomes a filter though which you see the world around you.

When stuck in the stress response, you can't think positively. Your attentional resources are focused on negativity. Fear is the focus, not friendliness. You are unable to make rational decisions. Choices are made on a short-term basis. Long-term consequences of choices can't be processed. If your fight-or-flight response is turned on continuously, you are in constant emergency mode and can only make short-term emergency decisions.

Nowadays, the same mechanism to prepare you to run from a tiger is switched on when you get stuck in a long line at the bank, are running late for work, dealing with a screaming child, or have to deal with your aggressive boss. Your body is preparing for a physical threat where none exists.

In modern society, rather than physically exerting yourself when your stress response is on, you're expected to control yourself. Waiting in a line, you're expected to just wait, no matter how late you are. When your boss makes unreasonable demands, you're expected to just listen, not fight or run away.

But fight or flight makes you more aggressive, hypervigilant, and over-reactive. This is what ultimately leads to photocopiers being kicked, road rage in major cities, and fights.

Balancing Your Nervous System: The Key to Managing Stress

I've mentioned that the stress response is hardwired into your brain and body to protect you from physical dangers. But fortunately, the ability to reduce your stress is also hardwired. Both of these systems work largely unconsciously. It's automatic and so is called the autonomic nervous system. But through mindfulness you can learn to spot when your stress response is activated and take action to reduce it.

This autonomic nervous system is made of two main parts:

1. **Sympathetic nervous system (stress response)**—the main function of this is to activate the fight-or-flight response.
2. **Parasympathetic nervous system (relaxation response)**—the main function is to activate the "rest and digest" system and to bring your body back to balance after the stress response has been triggered.

To show you just how physical the stress response is designed to be, look at the diagram on the next page.

Have you ever had a dry mouth when giving a presentation? Noticed your heart beating rapidly or breathing rate increase? Felt the need to visit the bathroom? All these are the physical effects of the stress response created by greater activity of your sympathetic nervous system. That's what people call "feeling stressed," and these effects are shown on the right-hand side of the diagram. Your emergency mode is on.

The actions of your stress response can be balanced by your

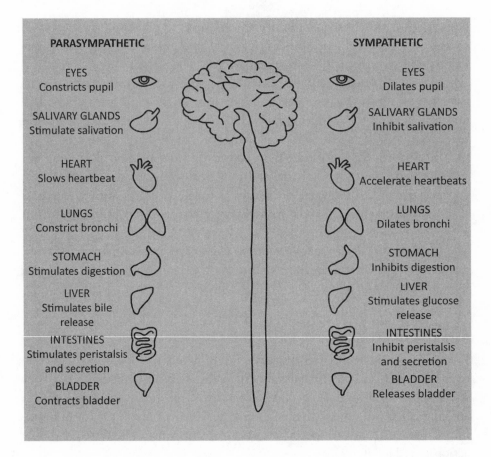

parasympathetic nervous system, which is your relaxation response. The relaxation response is sometimes called "rest and digest" mode because more of your resources are focused on digestion and immunity when activated. When you're stressed, your digestion doesn't work well. And over the long term, your immune system is severely affected too.

Although mindfulness is not a relaxation technique, one of the beneficial long-term side effects is relaxation. Mindfulness helps you notice when you're getting too stressed. Then you can do a short mindfulness exercise or meditation. This engages your prefrontal cortex, the wiser part of your brain. With access to your more rational brain, you can make better choices.

For example, let's say you're driving to see a new client. The roads are unfamiliar and narrow. It starts getting late, and you find the drive quite scary as there are no streetlights and others are driving so fast. You're running late and begin to feel stressed. You're mindful and notice your stress levels rising. So you stop by the side of the road and take a few mindful breaths. You start to relax a bit. You remember that driving safely is far more important than getting there on time. So you send a text to say you're running late and drive at a speed that is right for you, continuing to feel your breathing as you do so, rather than worrying. As shown in the seesaw diagram below, some activities engage your relaxation response and others engage your stress response. But these are not fixed.

Reflection

Consider the last time you felt really stressed. What changes did you notice in your body? How do they correspond to what you've discovered about the effects of the sympathetic nervous system?

GENERAL ADAPTATION SYNDROME: THE THREE STAGES OF STRESS

Walter Cannon discovered the fight-or-flight response in the 1920s, but it wasn't until 1936 that Hans Selye discovered the long-term response of the body to stress: the general adaptation syndrome. Essentially, Selye found that when something stressful happens, you go through three stages if the stress doesn't go away, shown in the graph on the next page. He found stress to be a major cause of disease because of the long-term chemical changes it wreaks on the body.

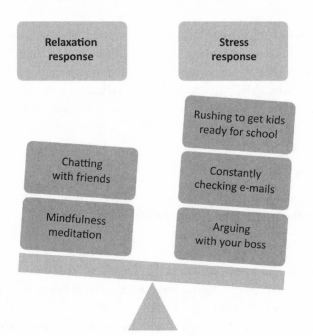

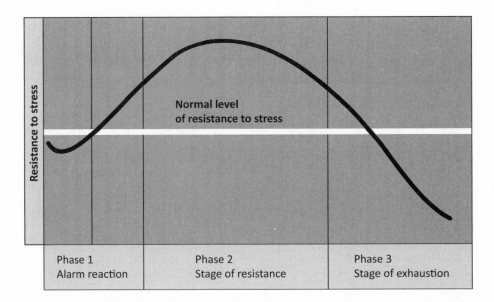

Stage 1: Alarm

In the alarm phase, you're in a state of shock. Imagine having lots of pressure at work and realizing that you can't get all the tasks done. You're initially less effective in your shock state. Your sympathetic nervous system is activated, and stress hormones are released into your blood system—the fight-or-flight response is working. If the stress is removed, you will return to a healthy balance.

At this initial stage, your body is working as it should, alerting and preparing you for a source of stress. And if you've been practicing mindfulness, you'll be aware that your stress response has been switched on. You can then take action to reduce the stress when you have time, by practicing a mindfulness exercise such as a mini body scan or mindful walking. This will help you get back into balance.

Stage 2: Resistance

If the stress continues to be present, however, or you experience additional stressors, you increase your fight against the challenge. This is the resistance phase.

At this stage, if you manage to cope with the stress in some way, your body can repair the damage caused by the alarm phase and your levels of stress hormones can return to normal. But problems begin if you don't have enough time to recover from this phase.

Mindfulness is very helpful to cope in Stage 2 as well; it can prevent you from reaching burnout. As you're under a significant amount of stress, you need to practice mindfulness meditations daily, if possible. Physically, the meditations give you the time required to feel the tension in your body, and paradoxically, that mindful awareness slowly begins to ease the tightness. Mentally, the mindfulness offers you the space to distance you from concerns and demands that may be driving the stress. Your relaxation response starts to get engaged, rebalancing your stress to a level that feels right for you.

If the stress continues, your immune system stops working well and you're less able to fight infection. Continued stress may eventually lead to Stage 3.

Stage 3: Exhaustion

The exhaustion phase occurs when the long-term stress does not go away. You can no longer resist the stressor because your coping resources have run out. Your levels of adrenaline, the stress hormone, are depleted. Selye found that animals, such as rats, just die in this state.

> "Once I understood the way stress can lead to resistance and finally exhaustion, my burnout made sense. I knew at that moment in the class, reducing my stress was now my number-one priority."

People call this burnout, adrenal fatigue, or stress overload. Ideas for identifying and dealing with it are in the box on page 144. At this point your stress levels are sky high and stay that way, and your health is at its greatest risk.

At this stage, you may not be ready to practice mindfulness because it's too hard for you to focus on anything. Once you've had some time to fully rest and recover, and after seeing a health professional, you can learn mindfulness to cope with stress more effectively.

Tales of Wisdom:
The Wise Sailor and the Intellectual Professor

There was once a professor traveling on a boat. He spotted an old sailor on the deck and decided to ask about marine science, a subject he had studied before. But the sailor said, "Sorry, I know nothing about marine science!" "You fool!" replied the professor.

The next day, the professor was on the deck looking at the stars. He thought the sailor must know about astronomy, to help with navigation. "I know absolutely nothing about astronomy," said the sailor. "You're a complete fool!" exclaimed the professor.

The next day, the professor felt the breeze against his skin. He thought the sailor must know about meteorology, the study of the weather. But alas, the sailor admitted he knew little about that science. "You complete idiot!" said the professor, vowing never to speak to the sailor again.

The next day, the boat faced rough winds and huge waves. The hull cracked and the boat started to sink. The sailor saw the professor and asked him, "Do you know how to swim?" "No!" exclaimed the professor. "Who's the fool now?" said the sailor as he dived in to swim to safety.

This story links well to managing stress mindfully. You can know all you want about the theory of dealing with stress, but until you put that knowledge into practice, it's of little benefit. Try out the meditations and learn to surf the waves generated by the stressors of life—the small effort will pay dividends.

Understanding Burnout

Burnout is a state of physical, mental, and emotional exhaustion due to long-term and excessive stress. You may be on the way to burnout if every day seems like a bad day, you're always tired, and you feel nothing you do makes a difference. Burnout is usually caused by overwork, but it can also result from not sleeping enough, lack of supportive relationships, perfectionism, or pessimism.

If you feel you're close to burnout, or are burned out, try the following tips:

- Start each day with mindfulness meditation or yoga.

- Eat healthily. Ensure you go to bed on time. Exercise a few times a week.

- Learn to say no, so you're setting your boundaries and not taking on too much extra work.

- Have some fun time every day or at least once a week. Do something that gets your creative juices flowing.

- Slow down the pace of your life.

- Get support from friends and family. You may feel you don't want to, but seek social support despite that—talking is very important.

Consider reevaluating your goals in life. Burnout is a sign that it's probably time to take a different approach.

Reflection

Are you currently suffering from the effects of long-term stress? How can you best take care of yourself over the coming weeks and months? If you think you're reaching the point of exhaustion, how can you make stress reduction your number-one priority?

Your body is designed to manage stress like a sprint, not a marathon. A mindful way through stress means finding small slots of time in your day to rest, recharge, or meditate—even a few deep mindful breaths will have a positive effect.

Occasional moderate levels of stress with periods of rest is healthy—just ensure enough time for recuperation.

Reflection

In 1914, 67-year-old inventor Thomas Edison's lab caught fire and burned down, destroying all his equipment and research. He lost $2 million in one night. Rather than think of the many negatives, he said, "There is great value in disaster. All our mistakes are burned up. Thank God we can start anew." That's a great example of turning distress into eustress. A few weeks later Edison delivered the first phonograph.

Consider a small or medium stress you're suffering from and write down how you could change your distress into eustress. Mindfully step back from your thoughts and see things from a bigger picture.

STRESS AND LIFE CIRCUMSTANCES

Different events in your life are bound to have a different effect on your stress. Moving to a similar neighborhood is not going to have as big an effect as a hostile divorce. The fewer major life events you experience in a relatively short period of time, the less likely you'll suffer the consequences of chronic stress.

Research Corner:
Stress Can Be Good for You—Discovering Eustress

Most people don't know that there are two types of stress: eustress and distress. Eustress is a positive form of stress, whereas distress is a negative form.

The actual stressor doesn't determine whether it would cause eustress or distress. Instead it depends on whether you see the situation as a positive challenge or a negative hassle.

Examples of eustress could be a roller coaster ride. If you look forward to the challenge of the experience, you'll have the stress response but feel positive about the experience. However, the same roller coaster ride is a source of distress if you think you won't be able to cope with the experience.

Even seeing stress itself as a positive experience is transformative. I'd like to share with you one of my favorite studies. In a major piece of research on almost 29,000 people over eight years, researchers Keller and colleagues at the University of Wisconsin–Madison found that people's attitude toward stress had a massive impact on how long they lived. If people saw stress itself in a positive way, believing it to be enhancing, they were among the least likely to die. However, those who believed stress was debilitating had a 43% increased risk of death. So think of stress as energizing or exciting rather than just harmful. Reading the paragraphs below may help you do this.

There is evidence that stress in short bursts actually boosts body function. In an interesting study in 2013 by Kirstin Aschbacher and colleagues at the University of California, two groups of women were asked to give a speech. The first group of women were already under chronic stress in their lives, but the other group were not. For the already stressed-out group, the extra stress caused extra damage in cells, as expected. But the next result surprised the researchers: the normally relaxed women were found to have less damage in their cells following the short burst of stress. A little bit of stress appeared to be helpful.

When you do physical exercise in short bursts and have periods of rest, your health improves. In the same way, short bursts of stress could have health benefits. Short bursts of stress release adrenaline, which increases alertness and awareness, just like a cup of coffee, as well as improving memory and sharpness of thought.

EXERCISE: Stressful Events in Your Life

On pages 148–149 is a list of 43 "stressful life events." Psychiatrists Thomas Holmes and Richard Rahe asked people to record how many of these life events they had experienced in the last year. Each event was given a score, and they found a link between the score and the likelihood that the person would suffer an illness.

Now you try it. Check off every life event you've experienced in the last year. If you experienced the event twice in the same year, enter two checkmarks. Then add up your score.

—— ∽

(TIP) If you found you got a high score, use this information as notification that you could make extra stress-reducing efforts. The practice of mindfulness could be particularly important for you at this time.

I've been fortunate in not having suffered too many changes in any one year. The most stressful was probably back in 2010, when a long-term relationship ended, I had some trouble with my boss, I changed my social activities, I published and launched my first book, I moved, I went traveling for a month, and quit my job all within a few months. Some of those changes were positive and refreshing rather than a burden—they were a source of eustress. However, I did get the flu and felt out of control. Without mindfulness things could have been much worse. I made sure I meditated every day, exercised regularly, kept a journal, and found time for some fun activities every week.

Reflection

So, what do you do if your score says you're at moderate or high risk of illness? The key is to minimize any further changes in your life if you have a choice. So if you've recently suffered the death of a close family member, perhaps you should hold off on relocating. If you've just retired and had a change in your financial position, it may not be advisable to also change your social and recreation activities right now. Write down what changes you can avoid making this year.

How Can Mindfulness Reduce Stress?

Consider Jodie. She was living with three roommates. One of them, Danielle, decided to let her boyfriend stay with her, even though this wasn't permitted in the lease. With an already overcrowded flat, Jodie felt annoyed when the boyfriend prevented her from using the bathroom in the morning and hogged

Stressful Life Events

Life Event	Life Change Units	✓
Death of a spouse	100	
Divorce	73	
Marital separation	65	
Imprisonment	63	
Death of a close family member	63	
Personal injury or illness	53	
Marriage	50	
Loss of job	47	
Marital reconciliation	45	
Retirement	45	
Change in health of family member	44	
Pregnancy	40	
Sexual difficulties	39	
Gain a new family member	39	
Business readjustment	39	
Change in financial state	38	
Death of a close friend	37	
Change to different line of work	36	
Change in frequency of arguments	35	
Major mortgage	32	
Foreclosure of mortgage or loan	30	
Change in responsibilities at work	29	
Child leaving home	29	
Trouble with in-laws	29	
Outstanding personal achievement	28	
Spouse starts or stops work	26	
Begin or end school	26	
Change in living conditions	25	
Revision of personal habits	24	
Trouble with boss	23	
Change in working hours or conditions	20	
Change in residence	20	
Change in schools	20	
Change in recreation	19	
Change in church activities	19	
Change in social activities	18	
Minor mortgage or loan	17	
Change in sleeping habits	16	
Change in number of family reunions	15	
Change in eating habits	15	
Vacation	13	
Christmas	12	
Minor violation of law	11	

Total: _____   (cont.)

From Holmes, T. H., & Rahe, R. H. (1967). The Social Readjustment Rating Scale. *Journal of Psychosomatic Research, 11*(2), 213–218. Copyright 1967. Reprinted with permission from Elsevier.

Score	Chance of Illness
Less than 150	Low to medium chance of illness in the near future
150–300	Medium to high chance of illness in the near future
Over 300	High to very high chance of illness in near future

the living room in the evenings. Her stress levels began to rise each day, but she ignored it. In the diagram below, she moved down the right-hand column.

Jodie confronted her roommate but wasn't sure she could handle the situation. Danielle was a lawyer and friends with the landlord. Following an argument with Danielle, and after the problem had gone on for several months, she started to get headaches, an upset stomach, and had trouble sleeping. The stress was affecting her.

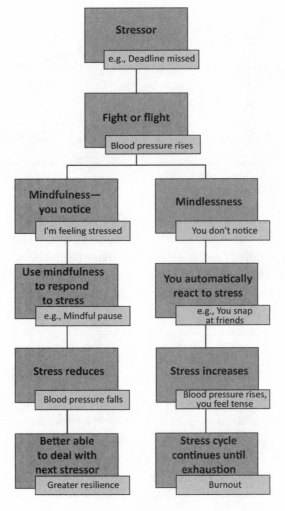

One of Jodie's friends guided her in a mindfulness meditation and taught her the mindful pause. Jodie was then better able to spot the signs of stress; tension in her shoulders and a locked jaw were her signs. Taking a mindful pause helped. But not for long. Jodie was using the pause just to relax and then going straight back to her normal way of thinking.

After reading more about mindfulness, Jodie started to take more responsibility for her own stress. Yes, Danielle wasn't being fair, but there was no point in making herself stressed and ultimately ill over the issue. With this attitude together with the mindfulness practice, she felt more confident. She asked herself what else she could do apart from argue with Danielle. In a calmer state, the solution was obvious: to contact the landlord. She gave him a call, and he immediately took action. Danielle's boyfriend was told to move out within a week, which he did. Danielle moved out with him.

Reflection

Consider something that's causing you stress at the moment. Think about how you are reacting to that stress. For example, are you working even harder, shouting at your partner, or trying to zone out through several hours of TV every night? At this stage, just write down how you're reacting. To observe this is mindfulness and is the first stage of making a positive change.

Tend and befriend explains why women are less likely to be aggressive compared to men when under stress—aggression being fueled by the fight-or-flight response. Women have a greater tendency to reach out to others when feeling stressed. This desire to be with others rather than immediately fight or flee may have evolved to protect children. Women in early history were the

Research Corner:
How Men and Women React Differently to Stress

The fight-or-flight response has been known about for many years. But the research has focused too much on males. There is now a new theory around: that women deal with stress through an additional and different mechanism, called "tend and befriend," first discovered by Shelley Taylor, a psychology professor at the University of California, together with her colleagues.

primary caregivers, and fighting or fleeing when in a stressful situation would put their children at greater risk of harm.

The reason for the difference in behavior is a hormone called oxytocin. Women have more oxytocin than men and so rather than have a fight or escape the stressful situation, the hormone encourages women to nurture and seek companionship. Research shows that when under stress, women seem to talk through their emotional experiences and explore the situation and what may happen next. Men prefer to react or flee—escaping the situation by going for a run, playing a sport, or watching television.

Obviously these are generalizations and every individual is different. But knowing these tendencies may help you better understand reactions to stress, both your own and those of friends and family.

Be mindful next time you see yourself getting stressed and notice whether you are engaging your fight-or-flight response or your tend-and-befriend response. If you feel excessive physical energy, you may benefit from a brisk mindful walk to ease your stress. If you feel like being with others, call or meet up with a friend for a chat. And be mindful of what they have to say—listen with mindful awareness.

Exploring Pleasant, Unpleasant, and Neutral Experiences

Life is made up of a wide variety of experiences that are automatically judged by your mind. In mindfulness, we classify experiences as pleasant, unpleasant, or neutral; see the diagram on the next page.

Over the last 2 weeks, you've been recording situations in your life that are pleasant or unpleasant and your associated thoughts, feelings, and bodily sensations. If you haven't done this, start this week and read this section after you've recorded them.

Pleasant experiences are those that you like and are enjoyable for you. Eating some chocolate, taking a warm bath, or feeling excited may be pleasant for you. Unpleasant experiences are those that you don't like. Eating spinach, waking up early, or feeling anxious may be unpleasant for you. Neutral experiences are those that you neither like nor dislike. For example, the color of the pavement, the coolness of a glass of water, or the feeling of your body against the back of your chair may be neutral for you—you zone out.

Over time, you become conditioned. You learn what's pleasant and seek to repeat the experience. And also learn what you find unpleasant and avoid it. This constant chasing after the pleasant and avoiding unpleasant or

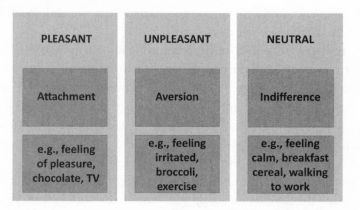

PLEASANT	UNPLEASANT	NEUTRAL
Attachment	Aversion	Indifference
e.g., feeling of pleasure, chocolate, TV	e.g., feeling irritated, broccoli, exercise	e.g., feeling calm, breakfast cereal, walking to work

neutral leads to a feeling of stress. You're in a state of mind of constantly running toward or away from experience.

Research in the field of positive psychology, the meticulous study of human happiness, has revealed many times that chasing pleasant experiences leads to a very fleeting happiness, whereas cultivating the practice of mindfulness meditation leads to a longer-lasting and deeper sense of well-being and peace.

> He who binds to himself a joy
> Does the winged life destroy;
> But he who kisses the joy as it flies
> Lives in eternity's sun rise.
> —WILLIAM BLAKE

Remember to keep this insight in perspective. I'm not saying all pleasures are bad or unhelpful—there's absolutely nothing wrong with having a delicious chocolate, a deep massage, or a long, hot bath. But evidence shows chasing sensual pleasures is not the royal road to a stress-free or happy life; it's just one way.

Mindfulness offers a way of releasing yourself from relentlessly chasing pleasant experiences and avoiding unpleasant or neutral ones. You simply need to be aware of the feeling of your daily experience and your experience in meditation. Each time you feel an experience is pleasant, unpleasant, or neutral, notice that as such. You'll begin to notice how your reaction to feeling dominates your everyday experience. In this way, you begin to step back from your conditioning. You notice your desire to cling or push away an experience. By watching the nature of your mind, with friendliness rather than self-judgment, you begin to break the chains of conditioning. As this happens, you are better able to enjoy the peace in the present moment.

(TIP) One of the best ways to let go of clinging to pleasant and running away from unpleasant experiences is to remember and notice that all experiences are impermanent. Using a sentence like "This will soon pass" helps you step back and ride the wave of the feeling without reacting to it.

Reflection

Look back at your pleasant and unpleasant events calendars. What patterns do you notice? For example, always avoiding the feeling of sadness by eating cookies (and feeling self-loathing after you do) or always seeking to talk to your partner even when he's too busy at work to chat (and feeling frustrated when he doesn't answer). Jot your observations down. In mindfulness, just noticing yourself nonjudgmentally is often enough to begin the shift in changing your habit patterns.

PRACTICE: **Mindful Yoga**

Audio track 9 or 10.

Now's the time to try some mindful yoga as part of this session. Do the mini (10-minute) or full (30-minute) yoga sequence using the audio or the instructions in Chapter 13.

PRACTICE: **Mindfulness of Breath and Body Meditation**

Audio track 13: 10 minutes.

Audio track 14: 20 minutes.

Having stretched your body, now you may feel ready for some mindfulness meditation in a seated posture. Remember, if your body is unable to sit for whatever reason, just choose whatever posture you can manage.

Your intention and attitude of mindfulness is more important than any-thing else. Listen to the audio track, which guides you through awareness of breath and body as described below.

1. If you can, sit in an upright, dignified posture on a chair, with your feet firmly on the floor and back relatively straight. Ensure you've switched off any potential distractions and it's relatively quiet; that's helpful for beginners. Set a timer if you're not using the accompanying audio.

2. Let go of ideas like trying to relax, wanting to calm your mind, or getting rid of tension. Instead, bring an attitude of accepting whatever arises, a sense of open, nonjudgmental receptivity to your moment-to-moment experience, as best you can.

3. Start the meditation with three deep, full breaths. If you can, breathe down into the base of your lungs, allowing your belly to gently expand on the in-breath and contract on the out-breath. If you can't feel this, try placing your hand around the area of your navel.

4. Now allow your breathing to return to its normal, natural rate. Allow your body to breathe on its own, rather than trying to do the breathing.

5. Each time your mind wanders and you've noticed that it has wandered, be pleased that you've noticed, rather than frustrated that your mind wandered. Bring your attention back to the phys-ical feeling of your breath around your nose, chest, or belly—wherever is easiest for you.

6. After 5 minutes or so, open your awareness to your body as a whole. Feel the sensation of your physical body as you sit here. Include both the pleasant and unpleasant sensations. Both those that feel warm or cool and those that have a sense of discom-fort. You may notice tingling, itching, heat, or some other sensa-tions. There may also just be the feeling of your body, alive and present.

7. Remember, the feeling of your breathing is also a bodily sensa-tion, so include the feeling of your body breathing too. Notice what effect your breathing has on your bodily sensations from moment to moment. Does your breathing increase or reduce muscle tension, or does it stay the same? Do other sensations stay exactly the same, or do they change from moment to moment?

8. After your time is up, gently bring your attention back to your surroundings. Take a few moments to notice this transition from

meditating to being in your everyday life. See if you can bring a sense of mindful awareness to the next moments of your day.

GOING DEEPER: When you feel a "difficult" sensation in your body, see if you can let go of all effort to get rid of the sensation. Just be completely attentive to the sensation itself—a complete feeling of acceptance to the sensation, knowing that it will eventually pass away, as all sensations do. You can even try to welcome the sensation, as if it's a feeling you actually like.

PRACTICE: Mindful Pause

You learned how to do the mindful pause in Week 2. At this stage of reading, I'd recommend you try that practice again. Remember, the aim is greater awareness of your state of body and mind, rather than a break or just relaxation.

Reflection: Discoveries about the Mindful Pause

1. What did you notice during your mindful pause this time around?

In my experience, people generally tend to fall into two categories. Either they regularly practice the mindful pause without an issue, or they find the practice really hard to do.

Those who have trouble don't have trouble with the technique. Rather, they have difficulty either finding the time or motivating themselves to do the practice. There's some sort of inner resistance.

The best way to overcome this resistance is to become aware of it in your body. Notice the sensations that the resistance brings. Feel the emotion of the resistance in your body and tune in to the thoughts that feed this resistance. Then take a few mindful, deep breaths and—guess what?—you're already doing a mindful pause by noticing the resistance.

The mindful pause reduces stress by switching off your habitual mind. You then step back from your usual thinking patterns, which may be feeding the stress. Awareness of your breathing begins to engage your parasympathetic nervous system and you begin to relax. You are then able to step back and see your stressor from a bigger perspective and might come up with a solution to deal with your stress.

2. How has the mindful pause been going for you over the last 2 weeks? What's working for you? What changes do you need to make to integrate the practice into your life—for example, setting a timer or putting the exercise in your calendar?

Mindfully Managing Stress FAQs

Q: Is it possible for me to be stressed and not actually know that I'm stressed?

A: I've been asked this question a few times. Yes, it is possible to be under stress without knowing. That's what being unmindful is all about. But through the practice of mindfulness, you become more aware of your body, emotions, thoughts, and actions, and so you're better able to notice when your stress levels get too high. You can then take appropriate action to manage that stress, such as by practicing the mindful pause.

Q: My mind is worrying all the time. How can I stop it?

A: One of the powerful effects of mindfulness is that it reduces rumination. This doesn't happen instantly. Gradually, you will notice your circular thoughts earlier and have a greater ability to step back from them. The key is not to fight the thoughts but to have a laid-back attitude and keep stepping back from them. Label them as "worry" and give attention to whatever you need to focus on.

Q: I felt quite tearful after the yoga. Is that okay?

A: Yes, that's fine. It's a good sign; it shows that you're practicing the yoga in a mindful way and are letting go of emotions that may have been suppressed and pushed out of your conscious awareness.

Q: I prefer to do the sitting meditation compared to the body scan. Can I do that instead?

A: I recommend you stick to the weekly home experiments. This way you overcome your mind's desires to do the mindful exercises you find pleasant and avoid the exercises that you find unpleasant. For example, I often find students don't like the body scan meditation for the first week or two, but after a while they really enjoy it.

Q: **I feel like I'm becoming less mindful as I go through this course! What's happening?**

A: This is a common response. Like most people, you may not have realized just how unmindful you normally are. By doing the mindful exercises and meditations, you're noticing just how easy it is to get lost in thoughts, emotions, and habits. So don't worry if you feel you're getting less mindful—in reality, the opposite is probably true. It's a bit like learning to ride a bike. It looks easy, but when you try, you just keep falling off. You may look as if you're getting worse, but actually, you're getting better.

Home Experiments: Week 4

Your home experiments are set out in the table on the next page, as usual.

Mindful Booster: Kindness

This week, try doing a very small favor for someone every day. You could send a friendly e-mail praising someone for his good work, offer a cup of tea or coffee to someone different at work, or help someone out with her project.

Your daily act of kindness doesn't have to take long. Even 5 minutes helping someone out not only makes you more mindful as you're stepping out of your usual routine, but also allows you to experience the act of giving. By limiting it to 5 minutes, you won't end up burdening yourself too much either.

These acts of kindness can be very beneficial both for you and for the recipient of your generosity. Research suggests acts of kindness can make you happier (because they release dopamine in your brain), healthier (because they drop your blood pressure due to the release of oxytocin), improve relationships (people like kind people), and most exciting of all, can help to spread kindness—your friends will be naturally inspired to perform an act of kindness. All these benefits will reduce your stress, so give it a try; spend up to 5 minutes a day doing an act of kindness for someone else. Find out more at *www.randomactsofkindness.org.*

Week 4

Day	Mini-Course	Full Course
1	Mini-body scan Mindful booster: kindness	Full body scan Mindful pause × 3 Mindful booster: kindness
2	Mini-mindfulness of breath and body meditation Mindful booster: kindness	Mindfulness of breath and body meditation Mindful pause × 3 Mindful booster: kindness
3	Mini-body scan Mindful booster: kindness	Full body scan Mindful pause × 3 Mindful booster: kindness
4	Mini-mindfulness of breath and body meditation Mindful booster: kindness	Mindfulness of breath and body meditation Mindful pause × 3 Mindful booster: kindness
5	Mini-body scan Mindful booster: kindness	Full body scan Mindful pause × 3 Mindful booster: kindness
6	Mini-mindfulness of breath and body meditation Mindful booster: kindness	Mindfulness of breath and body meditation Mindful pause × 3 Mindful booster: kindness

EIGHT

Week 5

Taking a Stand—Responding to Stress

The greatest weapon against stress is our ability
to choose one thought over another.
—WILLIAM JAMES

INTENTIONS

✦ *To discover four key ways of dealing with stressors.*

✦ *To understand how to relate to the thoughts and emotions that cause or arise from stress.*

✦ *To explore how to honor emotions that arise from stress so you find some relief.*

MINDFULNESS HAS become an incredibly important part of Fatima's life. She didn't like to sit down and purposefully meditate—she found that level of mindfulness incredibly difficult—but she willingly embraced mindfulness in her life. As someone who has struggled with anxiety for many years, she is no stranger to negative automatic thoughts that just won't go away.

In the past she found solace in planning for the future—escaping thoughts of the past and placing all her hopes and dreams in a place that didn't exist. This kind of thinking created a false idea of comfort because when the future did not happen—when her plans did not realize themselves—she felt lost.

Eventually she had to face the reality of her situation. What did she have? What could she possibly do now? She was terrified at the realization

159

that she no longer knew how to plan for her future. Initially she felt hopeless and worthless, but slowly she began to accept that *right now* she couldn't plan for the future and that was okay, because what she did have was *right now*. Once she knew this, once she had accepted this, she felt at peace because she knew that right now was all she needed. That was incredibly empowering, as it enabled her to pick herself up from a very dark and empty place and find comfort in the acceptance of *right now*.

Fatima handled her difficult emotions by living in the moment and accepting what she couldn't change. This viewpoint helped to dissipate her stress and anxiety.

Fatima also made a choice—a radical choice. A choice to look at her problems in a different way rather than be driven by the whims of the mind. And although meditation is what usually causes such a shift, just a more mindful way of looking at her problems helped. This chapter will look at how you can use a variety of ways to deal with stress and make yourself more resilient to future stressors too.

Reflection

You're halfway through: How's the course going?

Use the following questions to help you reflect on where you are right now with this mindfulness course. Jot your answers in your journal if you like.

1. What's going well for you?
2. Which practices have you tried?
3. Why are you doing this course? Remind yourself of your motivation.
4. Who is supporting you as you do this course? If the answer is no one, and you're finding the course challenging, whom could you ask? Even someone online or by phone could be useful.
5. Is there an area that you wish to improve on? If so, write it down. Focus on just one thing. What small steps can you take to improve that area?

TIP What's happened for you in the last 4 weeks is no indication of what'll happen next. In mindfulness, changes are not linear. You may not notice any significant changes so far, but that doesn't mean the next 4 weeks will be the same. Human beings are far too complex to be able to predict what will happen and when, so I urge you to try to keep an open mind and heart as you practice.

If you had trouble thinking about what's going well for you in the reflection exercise, consider that you've been reading this book, tried some of the meditations, tried a few of the home experiments, or any experience of living in the now. These are all examples of some progress, so you can record them as positive steps.

The one area that people often struggle with is actually doing the daily home experiments in mindfulness. If you're not doing them at all, consider what's getting in the way. Go back to Chapter 3 and reread the section on home practice. You may pick up some ideas to help rekindle your enthusiasm. Avoid self-criticism if you can—notice whether that's happening. And remember that noticing is a mindful act in itself. Just come back to right now, the present moment, and start afresh, as Fatima did. Look after the present moment and the future will look after itself.

This week, let's go straight into yoga and meditation practice. That helps to put you in a mindful state and makes you better able to focus on the theme of the session.

PRACTICE: Mindful Yoga

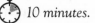

🕐 *10 minutes.*

🕐 *30 minutes.*

Audio tracks 9 and 10.

As usual, use the audio or instructions in Chapter 13 to do your mindful yoga practice today.

Reflection

1. What did you discover when exploring your edge in the yoga practice today?
2. What thoughts and emotions arose for you as you approached your edge in yoga?

3. Think about your life at home, at work, and how much you socialize and exercise. Are you pushing beyond the edge of your capacity? Or not challenging yourself at all? What choices are you able to make to redress the balance this week?

PRACTICE: Expanding Awareness Meditation

⏱ *10 minutes.*

⏱ *30 minutes.*

Audio tracks 15 and 16.

This week, you're going to practice the "expanding awareness" meditation. In other books on mindfulness, this is called the sitting meditation. The meditation is normally practiced in a sitting position, but that's not absolutely necessary. You could practice lying down, standing, or even walking (although that's tricky for beginners).

I'd recommend you do the meditation in a seated posture if you can, as it's usually easier to focus that way. As you may have been doing lots of body scan meditations lying down, now's a good chance to experiment with being in an upright posture and noticing how that affects your mindful awareness. Just be curious!

If you're doing the mini-course, spend just under 2 minutes on each part. Use the guided audio for 10 minutes. If you're doing the full program, spend about 5 minutes on each stage. Use the guided audio for 30 minutes.

Preparation

1. Eliminate any potential distractions.
2. Bring an attitude of friendliness and kindness toward yourself. Remember the reason you're practicing mindfulness and the importance of not trying too hard but being gentle with yourself.
3. Sit with an upright, dignified posture, on a chair that's right for you. Either close your eyes or softly gaze downward.

Stage 1: Breath

4. Take a few deep, full breaths. With each out-breath, have a sense of your body sinking a little deeper into your chair. Check your body for any obvious tensions and release them if you can. If you can't, that's fine. Just accept them as they are.

5. Now allow your breathing to be natural. Feel the physical sensation of your breath wherever you prefer. Notice how the sensation of the in-breath is different from the out-breath. Experience the natural rhythm of your breathing. Be aware of the brief pauses between each in- and out-breath. If your breathing pattern changes, notice that too.

6. As always, expect your mind to wander. When you notice that your mind wanders, whether it's for a few seconds or many minutes, just notice briefly what your train of thought was about and then very gently bring your attention back to your breathing. Remember: you can imagine your attention wanders like a puppy that wanders off a path. Bring your attention back with the same gentleness that you would pull the lead for the puppy to return to the path.

Stage 2: Bodily sensations

7. Open up your attention to all your bodily sensations. Be aware of how your focused attention on your breathing has the flexibility to open up to your body as a whole.

8. Notice how an open attention is different from a narrow, focused attention. If you can't seem to open your attention to your whole body, just do your best. With experience and practice you'll get better at it.

9. Be aware of your sensation of breathing as part of your bodily sensations. As you breathe in and out, notice what effect it has on your body. Be aware of the effect of your in-breath and out-breath. You may notice that the out-breath has more of a tension-releasing effect than your in-breath because your out-breath engages your parasympathetic nervous system (the relaxation response).

10. Keep your body and eyes still, as best you can. If you feel an itch or slight discomfort, see if you can tune in to that sensation without immediately reacting to the sensation. Become curious about the sensation by gently asking yourself questions like, "I wonder how the sensation's intensity increases or decreases as I observe and

breathe?" or "Can I feel this sensation with a sense of care and affection rather than reacting to it?" Or simply label it as "itch" or "pain" in your mind. If the discomfort increases and you feel you need to move, that's fine. You don't need to torture yourself in meditation. Simply be aware of how sensations in your body shift and change as you move from one posture to another. For example, if your back hurts, you may notice that pain, then gently stretch, feeling the muscles contract and relax, and again noticing the feelings in your back as you come back to sitting. The idea is to carry out the whole process consciously and mindfully rather than automatically and reactively.

Stage 3: Sounds

11. The next stage is to open up the attention even further. This time, turn your attention to sounds. Begin by noticing the sounds in the room you're sitting in and then open up to the sounds in the building as a whole and finally include the sounds outside too.

12. Normally, when you listen to sounds, you attach a meaning to them, classify them, and judge them with a like, dislike, or neutral attitude. This meditation is an opportunity to open your attention to all sounds and let go of your judgment or labeling. If your mind still labels the sound and judges it, that's fine; just notice that as a process of your mind from your perspective of awareness. For example, if you hear the sound of traffic and think, "That's traffic; I hate that noise," you can notice that as just a thought and actually listen to the sound of the traffic as it is.

13. Instead of feeling you need to reach out and grasp the sound, just allow the sounds to come to you. Be like a microphone, picking up sounds, no matter what they are, from all directions. This is really opening up your attention.

Stage 4: Thoughts

14. Now turn your attention to the thoughts in your head. You can either hear the thoughts in your mind or perhaps see images if you're more of a visual person.

15. Step back from the thoughts. Take the viewpoint of an observer, watching your thoughts happen, rather than doing the thinking, as if you don't actually do the thinking yourself, but watch your brain thinking by itself.

16. You may find it helpful to imagine clouds passing through the sky. Think of the open space as your awareness and the clouds as your thoughts. You can place your thoughts on those clouds and watch them come and go.

17. If you find you're not having any thoughts, that's okay. Notice the silence. You don't need to force yourself to have thoughts. If you find you're having lots of thoughts, that's okay too. Again, take the stance of an impartial observer.

18. This is not an easy process for most people. Just practice as best you can and see what happens.

Stage 5: Emotions

19. Turn your attention to how you're feeling emotionally, right now.

20. If you know what the emotion is, gently label it. For example, if you're feeling fearful, say "fearful" in your mind.

21. Bring a mindful attitude to your emotion. This means there's no need to judge your emotion as bad or criticize yourself for having the emotion. Instead, welcome the feeling if you can and notice as much as you can about it.

22. Notice where in your body you feel the emotion. If you find it in your body, be aware of the size and shape of the sensation. Notice your attitude toward the emotion (e.g., "I like it" or "I wish it would go away"). Make an inner space for the emotion rather than blocking the feeling.

23. Watch the emotion from the safe distance and security of your awareness. Awareness both heals emotions and helps you create distance from the emotion as an observer, so you don't get quite so swept up in rises and falls of an emotional roller coaster.

24. Feel the emotion together with your breathing to help soothe the sensation and anchor you in the now.

Stage 6: Open Awareness

25. Now practice an open attention—sometimes called choiceless awareness. In this process, you can open your attention and be aware of whatever is predominant in your awareness. This can be anything, from each of your senses to your breathing, your thoughts, or your emotions.

26. If you find your mind gets caught up in a train of thought, bring your

attention back to your breathing for a few breaths. Then try stepping back to your open awareness again. Just do the best you can.

27. When your time is up, bring the meditation gently to a close by taking a few deep, slow breaths and gradually opening your eyes and stretching your body. Bring a mindful awareness to whatever you need to do next.

GOING DEEPER: With experience, you don't need the guided audio. You could set a bell to ring every 5 minutes and go through each stage in silence.

Practical Ways of Responding to Stress

The mindful way through stress doesn't limit you to just using mindfulness meditation to cope with stress. Mindfulness is offered as the first step to give you greater choice—a chance to step back from any conditioned reactivity you may have to stress and gain the space to choose a better response.

Practicing mindfulness meditation and yoga, as you've been doing so far, is changing your brain so you're not so automatically reactive to your stress. But how do you cope with stress? What are your options? This week you'll be learning the different ways to handle stress.

> "I was really getting annoyed by the traffic noise in the class. Then we did mindfulness of sounds and it immediately stopped being annoying! That's a big breakthrough for me. The traffic, in my nonjudgmental awareness, sounded like the ocean."

COMMON UNHEALTHY WAYS OF REACTING TO STRESS

It's useful to be honest with yourself and clear in your mind about how you currently deal with stress. This may be your "shadow side," and you may not like what you see. But looking clearly at how things are at the moment is the best starting point with the mindful approach to stress.

Most common strategies for dealing with stress result in short-term relief. But unfortunately, in the long term they increase your level of stress.

Excessive smoking, drinking alcohol, and taking illicit drugs are common choices for people under too much stress. If you use these methods to calm yourself after a stressful day, begin by noticing your feelings when you do this. Just asking yourself how you feel before lighting a cigarette is an act of mindfulness. Be aware of thoughts like "I've *got* to have a drink" or "I'm *dying* for a smoke." Mindful awareness of your thought patterns can help to break the habit. Look out for any self-critical thoughts too—thoughts like, "I can never control myself" or "I'm an idiot to get into drugs."

Be as mindful as you can while using your habitual coping strategy. For example, if you smoke too much when you're stressed, try this: Feel the weight of the pack of cigarettes in your hand. Then slowly open the pack, remove the cigarette, and notice its weight and color. Really look carefully at it. Smell the cigarette. After a few minutes of careful mindful observation of your cigarette, light it. Hold the cigarette in your opposite hand to help you be less automatic and more mindful. Keep noticing your own thoughts and feelings. Sense the smoke entering your lungs. Fully notice any feelings of pleasure or disgust as you smoke. Feel each in- and out-breath. Be aware of your physical tension or relaxation. Research has found taking 15–30 minutes to mindfully smoke one cigarette greatly increases your ability to reduce the amount you smoke in the weeks that follow such an exercise.

There are other ways you may be dealing with stress too, not just cigarettes or alcohol. Perhaps you start eating loads or eat far less. Maybe you're constantly procrastinating, surfing the Web, or watching TV when overwhelmed with stress. Or perhaps you get really busy, using work as a distraction from stress. Avoiding friends and family is another common behavioral pattern.

No matter what you end up doing, be as mindful as you can, even while engaging in the unhelpful habit. If you know you're avoiding your friends because you feel really stressed, notice the emotion that's driving you to do that. Allow yourself to slowly open up to the feeling of wanting to avoid others. Feel a few breaths together with the emotion. Notice how tense or tight your body feels.

Mindfulness and compassion are just as important when you make the wrong choice—learning to be kind to yourself, to forgive yourself (see Chapter 10) makes it more likely you'll make a better choice next time. Work by Chris Germer from Harvard Medical School and Kristin Neff from the University of Texas have found this to be true in their work with self-compassion—being self-compassionate lowers stress and helps you make better choices.

As best you can, avoid self-criticism and replace those thoughts with curiosity and acceptance. Say to yourself:

> "I'm going through a tough time at the moment. That's why I'm coping with the stress in this way. No one's perfect when it comes to dealing with stress. Let me be kind and understanding toward myself."

(TIP) Write this statement down on a little card and carry the card with you or put it on a smartphone you have with you, if you think it would work for you. Refer to the card or phone whenever you feel your stress rising.

I'm a work in progress, just like everyone else. I sometimes react to stress by eating more, procrastinating, surfing online, and avoiding my friends and family instead of calling them. Knowing this can help me watch out when I react in this way, and after taking a few mindful breaths, or more, I can make a better choice. It's not always easy, and sometimes that choice can take some time.

FINDING HEALTHY WAYS TO RESPOND TO STRESS

If your current strategies for dealing with stress aren't working, or you feel you're not dealing with your stress at all, don't worry. You're now going to discover a variety of different ways of managing stress. Your job is to try them out and see what works for you. Everyone is different, and so each person will use a different combination of stress management approaches that works for him or her.

Mindfulness lies at the heart of all the various ways of managing stress. When you're under stress, you need to be aware (mindful) that your stress levels are too high and then find a space to make a wise choice as to what's the best option for you. Always start your stress management strategy with a small, mindful exercise; the mindful pause is a great idea. Even one full, deep, conscious breath can work wonders as a starting point for making a mindful choice.

THE FOUR A'S OF STRESS MANAGEMENT

A popular model to remember the range of ways to reduce stress is the four A's of stress management: avoid, alter, accept, or adapt (see the diagram on the next page). Avoid and alter are about changing the actual stressor itself—the cause of your stress. That's the first thing to try. You may be able to cut out the stress altogether. Accept and adapt are about changing your *response* to the stressor. One more thing you can do is to try to maintain a healthy lifestyle; see the box on page 171.

Avoid the Stressor

Often, you don't actually need to deal with the stress. There are ways of eliminating the stressor in the first place. For example, when I was offering too many coaching sessions to my clients, my workload became too heavy. So I

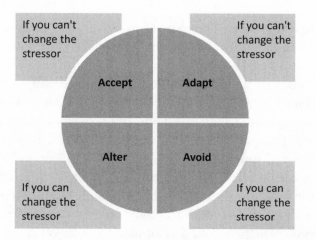

learned to limit the number of people I see every week to give me more time for writing and other work. Another example: I've had a couple of friends in the past who started off by being very friendly and nice but ended up being overly demanding and causing far more stress than I needed. Although it's never nice to have to end a relationship, after some time agonizing over the decision, I opted to distance myself from them.

Here are a few suggestions, but before you decide where to cut stress by cutting out stressors, try to determine whether the change you're considering will exert even more stress than the original obligation. Saying no, for example, might seem like it will be a huge relief—until you find yourself losing sleep over who will take over the task. Mindfulness can help you stay aware of and even anticipate your reactions to changes.

- **Say no.** Just because someone asks you to do something, you don't have to agree. If you do that, you'll end up with too much to do in too little time. The result is almost always stress.
- **Manage external factors.** If e-mail causes you stress, check it less often. If cooking is stressful for you, eat out from time to time. If commuting is stressful, see if you can work from home.
- **Stay away from negative people.** If certain people make you feel more stressed, just spend less time with them or end the relationship.
- **Reduce your to-do list.** Cut your daily tasks down to only the highest-priority items.

Alter the Stressor

If you can't cut out the cause of your stress altogether, you may be able to modify it, making it smaller and easier to handle. Here are some ideas:

- **Manage your time.** The cause of your stress may be having too much to do and too little time. Remember that Da Vinci, Einstein, and JFK had the same 24 hours that you do—you probably can find ways to be more efficient. I achieved better time management in the following way: First I became more mindful of what I was doing every 30 minutes by writing down what I was doing and how efficient I was being (e.g., writing e-mails 7/10 efficient, writing chapter 5/10 efficient). Then I discovered times in the day I was most efficient and times when I just needed a break. I shifted my most challenging and high-priority tasks in my most efficient time block (usually mornings) and left other errands for the afternoon. You could give this approach a try.
- **Express feelings to find a solution.** If you let others know how you feel about your situation, they may have a way of finding a solution. Be mindfully present with your emotions and express them gently when you can. Several research studies show writing things down in a journal can help too.
- **Set boundaries.** You need to be mindful of how much time and energy you're going to put into each task. If it's open-ended, other people can take advantage of you. Let other people know where the limit is, with both politeness and firmness.
- **Make compromises.** Often you can't fully get your own way. For example, agree to take your son to football only if he cleans his room every week—that's one less thing for you to do.

Accept the Stressor

One key to stress management is knowing what you can control and what you can't. If you can't control the stressor, you need to find a way to accept what's happening. Here's how:

- **Practice mindfulness meditation.** By meditating, your wisdom grows as you see how thoughts and feelings are constantly in flux. You learn to accept these changes rather than struggle to control them. This ability to accept is then translated to other areas of your life.
- **Let go of grudges.** Forgiving isn't always easy, but it can save years of unnecessary stress. By forgiving, you let go of grudges that usually cause you much more pain than the other person. And remember that forgiving doesn't mean what the other person did was right or fair. Forgiveness is for you, not for them.
- **Manage your inner control freak.** To manage stress, you need to be

clear about what you can control; you need to be able to accept the rest. If you don't accept what you can't control, that's a recipe for a stress-filled life.

- **Express your feelings.** By verbalizing your feelings to others, your brain turns down your stress response and you feel better. Sharing your problems helps to take a weight off your shoulders and makes acceptance a little easier.

Adopt a Healthy Lifestyle

Beyond the four A's for managing your stressor, it's a great idea to adopt a healthy lifestyle. Here are a few tips:

- **Exercise.** Aim for 30 minutes of physical activity, 5 days a week. Even a brisk walk counts. Make your exercise mindful by paying attention to your bodily sensations, your breathing, or your senses.

- **Socialize.** Try spending time with others regularly. It'll often make you feel calmer and keep things in perspective. Practice mindful listening by letting go of your own judgments while listening to your friend.

- **Balanced diet.** Taking the time and effort to eat well will make you feel good about yourself and boost your energy and resilience against stress. And if you end up eating a package of cookies, see if you can be kind to yourself rather than berate yourself. Self-compassion is an important, mindful attitude.

- **Sleep.** Aim for 7½–9 hours a night if you want optimal health. If you can't do this during the week, catching up on the weekend doesn't actually work that well. If you struggle to sleep, try using the body scan meditation at night to see if that helps.

- **Have fun every day.** Doing things just for fun isn't a luxury, but necessary for your sanity. Watch your favorite comedy, take a quiet stroll in nature, play a sport, or go to a party—whatever works for you. Be mindful while you're there rather than playing on your phone to fully take the experience in.

- **Relaxation.** Having a hot bath, getting a massage, savoring a delicious meal, and doing some light gardening are some of the many ways you could relax. And many of these activities can be enhanced by being mindful of them.

Adapt to the Stressor

Acceptance isn't the only way of dealing with stressors that you can't control. You can also change your mind-set—your attitude toward the stressor. This is called adapting to stressors. Here are some key attitude shifters that I often use:

- **See problems as opportunities.** Life will always be filled with problems. See them as challenges and opportunities and you'll feel less stressed and more excited.
- **Be grateful for what's going well.** Your brain isn't designed to remember positive events. So make a daily effort to consider what's going well in your life. Small things like a meal on the table, a view of some trees outside, and your ability to walk are all fine. If your boss is causing you stress, remember to be grateful for aspects of the work you enjoy—the salary, benefits, or colleagues.
- **Lower your standards.** Do you set yourself very high standards? Have a tendency toward perfectionism? Find out ways to reduce this way of living to make life less stressful and more productive and enjoyable.
- **Think big picture.** Consider whether your stressor will be an issue in a year's time. And how important is it, compared to the rest of your life? Practice stepping back to see things in perspective.

Reflection

Bring to mind a source of stress for you at the moment. Which of the four A's most appeals to you to respond most effectively to that stress? Try it out and write down what effect it had on your stress levels.

Differentiating Thoughts and Feelings

You've discovered some ways of managing stress. But you may not be clear about the difference between thoughts and feelings. For example, you may say:

"I feel useless."
"I feel pathetic."
"I feel ugly."

These are not emotions but thoughts. Examples of emotions include happiness, sadness, anger, boredom, fear, joy, excitement, and despair.

It's important to distinguish between thoughts and emotions because you can question your thoughts but not your feelings. Thoughts are sentences in your mind. You can step back from them, question them, or see them as simply sounds that are passing in your mind. Emotions are different. They are an inner experience usually including a bodily sensation. They are an experience that can't be questioned.

Ugliness is not a feeling—it's a thought. You probably feel sad and think, "I'm ugly." You can now question the thought. There may be many times when people found you beautiful. You may feel sad, but when you question the thought, the intensity of the feeling dissipates.

Thoughts affect emotions, and emotions affect thoughts. They interact with each other, together with sensations in your body. For example, when you feel lonely, you may start thinking, "I'm a loser," and your body may feel a bit weaker. This may then result in your feeling sad, and then you may think, "What's wrong with me?" and so on. The good news is you can make a positive difference. By labeling the emotion and changing your relationship to your thought, you start to take greater control of your emotions. The key way to shift your relationship to thoughts is explained next.

THOUGHTS ARE JUST THOUGHTS

Try saying the following sentence in your head:

"I'm a pink banana."

You obviously don't believe that to be true, but why not? After all, you had it as a thought in your head. As you know, just because you have a thought in your head doesn't make it a fact.

But what if you had the following thought in your head:

"I'm useless."

That's just another thought. But you may be more inclined to believe it, especially after a day when everything seemed to go wrong. (We talked about the negativity bias, which makes us all more inclined to interpret things negatively than positively, in Week 2.) If that thought has popped into your head before, or any other negative sweeping statement about yourself, your body's stress response would turn on. But if you see the thought for what it is—just another thought—then it can have far less power over you.

Research Corner: De-stress Your Brain by Labeling

In mindfulness, labeling emotions means stating in your mind what your experience is. For example, if you're feeling angry, you state in your mind, "I'm feeling angry" or simply "angry."

In 2007, J. David Creswell and colleagues from UCLA wanted to see whether this labeling had any effect on the brain, so they took a group of 27 people and showed them images of faces that were angry or fearful while in a brain scan. These images usually create the stress response in the brain, which includes increased activity in a part of the brain called the amygdala.

When the participants labeled the emotion with the word *angry* or *fearful*, they found that the activation in the amygdala reduced. Instead, they activated a part of the brain called the right ventrolateral prefrontal cortex, which is thought to help us deal with emotions and manage behavior. If they labeled the faces with any other name, they didn't get the same effect.

The study also found those who were more mindful had greater activity in the prefrontal cortex as a whole—the part of the brain intended to manage emotions, do problem solving, and make wise choices.

So, if you're feeling a difficult emotion, label it in your mind. Doing so can help you reduce your stress response and the intensity of the emotion. You could also write the emotion down in a journal or talk to a friend about how you're feeling to verbalize your emotions.

I know for me personally, thoughts were the cause of a lot of stress. When I taught my first lesson as a science teacher, I didn't think I was a good teacher at all. My hands were shaking, and each sentence I spoke was meticulously planned. I was so nervous while demonstrating a laser that I accidentally left the laser switched on and pointing toward the class! Luckily no one was hurt. But what was the cause of my stress? It was thoughts in my head saying things like "You can't teach," or "You're going to lose control of the class." And at first I believed those thoughts to be true. It was only after practicing mindfulness that I learned the adage:

Thoughts are simply thoughts—not necessarily facts.

This insight did change my life. I know that sounds cliché, but it did. I no longer believed the thoughts in my head have to be true. They are just that: thoughts. I learned to watch my thoughts and let them go, or question them, and went on to become a successful schoolteacher for 10 years! If I had believed those negative thoughts about myself all those years ago, I would have stopped teaching before I had really started.

You may argue, what if the thoughts are actually true? To help you check whether a thought is true, ask yourself the following question:

"Can I be 100% sure this thought is a fact?"

If you have any doubt about the thought's validity, just see it as merely a passing thought for the time being, especially if it's a judgmental thought.

Thoughts to watch out for are sentences with the words *always, never, should*, or *must*. They indicate that you're thinking in absolutes, which is rarely the reality. Life is not black or white. For example, when I have a heavy workload, my brain sometimes thinks, "I must finish this"—the strong word creates an unnecessary extra pressure on my mind. Here are some more examples of thinking in extremes:

"I always mess up."
"I should be working."
"She must get there on time."
"He never does anything nice for me."

Reflection

The next time you think a negative thought about yourself, follow it by saying, "Thoughts are just thoughts." Then take a mental step back from the thought. Record what effect this has.

AWARENESS AS A CONTAINER FOR EXPERIENCE

One of the ways of seeing thoughts as merely thoughts rather than facts is to learn the concept of awareness as a huge container for experience. In this way you're able to see thoughts, emotions, and all other experiences in a larger and more spacious way.

When I was first taught meditation, I found the process so exciting that I spent as much time as I could meditating. Sometimes I would meditate for hours. I was studying for my university degree in chemical engineering at the time and remember meditating instead of revising for my exams! Anyway, in those extended meditation sessions, I sometimes had a very unusual experience. The physical sensation in my body completely dissolved. I knew I was sitting there of course, but the physical limitations of my body disappeared. It was like my body wasn't there. Simultaneously my mind was completely open, and if I had a thought, it was completely clear in my consciousness and didn't hook me into a train of thought at all. The feeling was deeply restful, peaceful, and lasted for 10 minutes or so at a time, and when I ended the meditation my brain felt extremely wide awake, serene, and energized. I felt like I was resting in pure awareness itself.

> "I never felt the deep peace in the meditations that some others did. I thought I was doing it wrong. But then, one day, while in the shower, I felt happy for no reason. Just happy to be alive. I hadn't felt that for years. I knew it was the meditation that caused that."

Awareness is like a container for all experiences. All my senses, my thoughts and my emotions, my hopes and desires, dreams and fears are held within awareness. Without awareness, they have no existence.

Through regular mindfulness meditation, you'll discover this for yourself. Awareness is both lighting up all your experiences in the meditation and making you the observer of the experience rather than the experience itself. It's not an objective experience, but a subjective one. It can be described as "being," "presence," "aliveness." I like to simply think of it as pure awareness and that it lies at the heart of my being—always available and always free.

There are three main advantages of becoming familiar with awareness as a container for experience:

- You are able to step back from everyday negative experiences more easily. Therefore they don't cause so much stress.
- You are able to live with greater equanimity and therefore peace, because the rise and fall of thoughts and emotions are just seen as little events in the vast container that is awareness.
- You can feel satisfied with yourself just as you are. You don't need to keep striving to improve yourself, as your true nature is already pure and perfect just as it is.

The concept of a container is just an analogy. Some would say it's not even a container, as that creates a limit. You could think of awareness as open space, pure potential, or like the ocean, with the waves at the surface representing your thoughts and emotions and the calm and peacefulness at the bottom of the ocean.

Most people intuitively know there is a sense of deep peace within them. Meditation offers a way to dive down and access those precious inner resources and rise up refreshed and renewed.

(TIP) Avoid trying to chase any kind of "experience" in meditation. All experiences have a beginning and an end. Mindfulness is about letting go of all experiencing and just practicing the various exercises. Even if you do happen to experience "pure awareness," acknowledge it, enjoy it, and then turn your attention back to the meditation practice once the experience passes. Live in the moment rather than trying to relive past experiences.

Mindfulness and Resilience

Resilience is the process of effectively coping with adversity—it's about bouncing back from difficulties. The great thing about resilience is that it's not a personality trait; it involves a way of paying attention, thinking, and behaving that anyone can learn.

World-renowned neuroscientist Richard Davidson has found evidence that mindfulness does increase resilience, and the more mindfulness meditation you practice, the more resilient your brain becomes. The emotional soup that follows a stressful event can whip up negative stories about yourself or others that goes on and on, beyond being useful. For example, if you have an argument with your partner before leaving for work, you can end up replaying that conversation all day, which continues to proliferate anxiety or low mood far more than is necessary. Mindfulness reduces this rumination and, if practiced regularly, changes your brain so that you're more resilient to future stressful events.

There are several key aspects of resilience:

- Positive relationships—this is the most important factor.
- The ability to make plans and take action to solve problems.
- The capacity to manage difficult emotions—mindfulness is an important aspect here.
- Effective communication skills.

Here are five ways to build resilience:

1. **Nurture relationships.** Have a range of positive, supportive connections within and outside your family. If you don't, take steps to improve the situation. Join a club, local group, religious organization, volunteer group, or an evening class.

2. **Find meaning in difficulties.** When faced with adversity, see if you can discover some positive way in which you've dealt with the challenge. People often report improved relationships, greater spirituality, or appreciation of life in the face of great difficulties.

3. **Be optimistic.** Use mindfulness to shift your attention from negative rumination to more positive thoughts about the future. Hope and optimism is a choice. Avoid seeing crises as insurmountable. You can't change the fact that very stressful events happen, but you can learn to change your response to that. The tiniest of changes counts, and meditation can help.

4. **Be decisive.** Make decisions and take action rather than hoping things will get better one day. If you're not good at this, read about how to improve this skill or ask a trusted friend to help. Not making a decision is in itself a decision.

5. **Accept that change is part of living.** Expect things to change and adversity to occur, rather than pretend all will always be well. Change is part of life. Your goal is to cope effectively rather than avoid loss or pain.

When it comes to resilience, flexibility is the name of the game. Discovering ways to adapt to the changes that life throws at you makes you more able to cope.

> ## Reflection
>
> What simple action can you take to begin increasing your resilience? It can be as simple as picking up the phone and making a call every day.

Honoring Emotions

One powerful way of managing difficult emotions that arise in adversity is to honor all your emotions. It's okay to have emotions—all emotions. In fact, it's essential. The wide spectrum of emotions that humans experience is there for a reason. Research continues to show that people who use emotion and reason together make the wisest decisions. Reason can't operate effectively without emotion.

Emotions are like messengers. They exist to tell you something. When you experience a pleasant emotion, you're being informed to move toward something. When you feel an unpleasant emotion, you're being advised to move away. At their extreme, these emotions help you keep your hand out of a flame (fear) and spend time with other people (love). An emotion like depression may indicate you are criticizing yourself too much. The feeling of anger may be telling you someone is stepping beyond your boundaries.

The first step toward honoring emotions is to actually notice them. If you're feeling sad, notice where you feel the emotion in your body, as precisely as you can. The more you practice locating the feeling, the more mindful you become. Labeling the emotion in your mind is helpful too. Meticulous research by world-renowned expert on emotion Paul Ekman, across different cultures, found that there are only six core emotions: happiness, anger, fear, sadness, disgust, and surprise. Learning to identify these emotions is an important part of honoring them.

The second step is to stop judging your emotions. You may think of some emotions as good and others as bad. Or you may see all emotions as bad and irrational. That's just not true. Emotions have evolved within humans over thousands of years for a reason. Judging yourself for having certain emotions just leads to a negative feedback loop locking you deeper into the emotion itself.

The third step, and one of the most powerful ways of honoring your emotions, is to discover how to be compassionate toward yourself and your emotions. This acts like an antidote to berating yourself, which so many of us do, often unknowingly.

Consider this; How would you treat your friends when they were upset? Would you criticize them for feeling sad, or would you listen to them? Would you offer them a hug or push them over? Of course, you would seek to be kind to them. Well, try doing the same today with your feelings, especially the ones you normally judge as bad or wrong. If that doesn't feel comfortable for you, just try today, as an experiment. When you feel sad, say to yourself something like, "It's okay to feel sad. It's natural. Let me show kindness to the sadness. Let me hold the feeling with gentleness—with respect." Try placing your hand softly on the area in your body where you feel the emotion, as you would on a friend who was hurt—with care and affection. Feel the emotion together with your breathing. Remember that this feeling is universal; all human beings suffer with this feeling too.

> "I wish they had taught me about acceptance at school. I've been resisting emotions all my life, and it has caused me to break down. Now I accept. I've stopped fighting with my reality. For me it's the best way to be with emotions."

Tales of Wisdom:
Even the Dalai Lama Was Surprised

When the Dalai Lama was at a meeting with Westerners, meditation teacher Jack Kornfield and others explained how self-hatred, shame, and self-criticism were among the biggest challenges that people faced. It took the Dalai Lama 10 minutes of discussion with the translator to understand the concept of self-hatred. When he understood the meaning, he was genuinely shocked. In the Tibetan tradition, there is no word for self-hatred because it didn't exist in that culture. Whatever the reason, self-hatred is not helpful, and self-compassion is the solution. As the Dalai Lama responded, "But every being is precious!" Self-compassion and mindfulness can help you see yourself as just as precious as anyone else—which you are.

Reflection:
Discoveries from Week 4

Here's a chance for you to reflect on your experiences from the week that's just gone.

MINDFULNESS OF BREATH AND BODY MEDITATION

How did you find the mindfulness of breath and body meditation practice? Did you manage to adopt a seated posture for that meditation? If so, how did you manage any aches or pains arising in your back or other parts of your body?

Don't worry if you found it painful; that's often quite common, as most people aren't used to sitting upright and still for long periods of time. With practice, your back will strengthen and you'll find it easier.

MINDFUL BOOSTER: KINDNESS

Did you remember to do an act of kindness every day, or at least a couple of times during the week? If so, what effect did the action have on your state of mind? Is it something you'd like to do more regularly?

Responding to Stress FAQs

Q: **I'm losing enthusiasm for the mindfulness practice. Is that normal? Should I stop meditating?**

A: Around Week 3 or 4 of the course, people often experience a dip in motivation. The initial excitement of discovering a new tool to manage your stress may have diminished, and your romantic ideas of meditation as being your quick-fix method to eliminate stress may have been popped like a balloon. But don't stop. This is entirely normal. This is where the work starts. Keep going—there's lots more to discover and enjoy.

Q: **Why do I keep putting meditation off when I know it's good for me?**

A: This seems to be a common phenomenon for many people. Stopping what you're doing to be mindful or to meditate may go against all your upbringing, conditioning, and cultural norms. So there's bound to be some resistance. Rather than fighting the resistance, feel it. Notice what thoughts are driving this behavior. What feelings prevent you from meditating? As soon as you notice that, you're already being mindful.

Q: **I keep switching between the mini and full course. Is that okay?**

A: That's fine. You can do whichever one suits you in any one week. The shortest of practices is better than nothing at all.

Home Experiments: Week 5

This week's main home experiment alternates between the expanding awareness mindfulness meditation and either the body scan or yoga. You can choose whatever you feel is right for you. Remember to use the table on pages 182–183 to find out what you need to be practicing this week, and keep recording your findings in your journal. Here are some details about the other home experiments for this week.

Mindful Booster

This week's mindful booster is practicing gratitude. There is now lots of evidence to suggest that counting your blessings not only lowers stress but raises your level of happiness, improves relationships, and even helps you sleep. You could practice gratitude every day by noting a few things in your journal, thinking about them as you drift off to sleep, or sharing what you're grateful for with a friend or your partner every night during dinner. Use whatever approach you like to reflect on what you're grateful for every day. Think of different things or people to be grateful for every day to keep the process fresh.

Difficult Communications Record

Next week, you will be exploring mindfulness in communication. To prepare you for this, one of your recommended weekly tasks involves recording your difficult communications.

Answer the following questions every day in which you have a difficult communication. The communication could have been in person, on the phone, or even by e-mail. Effective communication is so important for managing stress—it's worth the few minutes it takes every day to try this. Even if this process leads to one insight, it's time and effort well invested.

1. Whom were you communicating with?
2. What was it about?
3. How did this communication come about?
4. What did you want from the communication?
5. What did you get from the communication?
6. What did the other person want?
7. What did the other person get?
8. What were your thoughts, feelings, and body sensations then?
9. What are your thoughts, feelings, and body sensations now?

Week 5

Day	Time	Mini-Course	Full Course
1		Mini-expanding awareness meditation Mindful booster: gratitude	Full expanding awareness meditation Mindful pause × 3 Difficult communications record Mindful booster: gratitude

Day	Time	Mini-Course	Full Course
2		Mini-body scan or mini-yoga Mindful booster: gratitude	Full body scan or full yoga Mindful pause × 3 Difficult communications record Mindful booster: gratitude
3		Mini-expanding awareness meditation Mindful booster: gratitude	Full expanding awareness meditation Mindful pause × 3 Difficult communications record Mindful booster: gratitude
4		Mini-body scan or mini-yoga Mindful booster: gratitude	Full body scan or full yoga Mindful pause × 3 Difficult communications record Mindful booster: gratitude
5		Mini-expanding awareness meditation Mindful booster: gratitude	Full expanding awareness meditation Mindful pause × 3 Difficult communications record Mindful booster: gratitude
6		Mini-body scan or mini-yoga Mindful booster: gratitude	Full body scan or full yoga Mindful pause × 3 Difficult communications record Mindful booster: gratitude

NINE

Week 6

Mindful Communication

*The single biggest problem in communication
is the illusion that it has taken place.*
—GEORGE BERNARD SHAW

INTENTIONS

✦ *To explore mindful communication.*

✦ *To practice applying mindfulness in different ways to listen deeply and speak effectively.*

✦ *To discover the roles of emotions and stress in communication and how to manage them.*

THIS IS the story of Hiroto, one of my readers and followers online.

Hiroto depended on his partner for his happiness. Whenever he felt annoyed or frustrated about anything, he took it out on her, and more often than not, that resulted in an argument. If he was not happy, he blamed his girlfriend. This seemed entirely reasonable to him. He didn't help with the cleaning in the house much, and she hardly ever cooked.

One of his friends had recently completed a course in mindfulness and kept raving about it, so Hiroto decided to give it a try, partly out of curiosity. He took to it like a duck to water, and although it reduced his stress, it did this in a way that was totally unexpected.

Hiroto's perspective on life and his relationship has improved in different ways as a result of mindfulness. He's now much less reliant on his partner for his happiness. He's less focused on her and more focused on cultivating his own well-being. Hiroto now takes a moment to look

184

mindfully within himself when feeling frustrated. This makes him feel better. How does he do this? By spotting negative thought patterns and tendencies to avoid difficult emotions early, and then practicing a short mindful exercise, which helps to dissipate these negative habits. Before mindfulness, Hiroto dealt with feelings of anxiety by arguing with and blaming his partner. Negative thought patterns included habitually thinking, "Why is she not making me happy?" or "Why is she stressing me out? It should feel relaxing to be with her," followed by thoughts and statements of how she should do this or that.

His relationship feels much more relaxed and positive now. Hiroto's new way of being has taken pressure off his partner now that he is more mindful. He seems to be more relaxed and is now talking about having children together, whereas before he was cautious about committing to the relationship.

Hiroto's change occurred when he discovered a greater awareness of his own thoughts and behavior. The next step was not to immediately react to his negative thought patterns and difficult emotions. He gradually acquired the ability to step back from thoughts and emotions and choose a healthier action instead of engaging in his usual habitual patterns of reactivity.

Reflection:
Exploring Your Difficult Communications Record

Before we dive into more theory this session, take a few moments to look at your difficult communications record, which you filled in last week if you did the home experiments for the full course.

The purpose of the difficult communications record was to give you an opportunity to see any patterns in your thoughts and feelings and body sensations in difficult conversations that you had throughout the week. Did you notice any patterns?

When I filled the record in myself, I noticed that my most difficult communications were with a friend. A close family member of his had just died, and I needed to call him. Noting my experience helped me see that I had some feelings of anxiety before and during the call and felt it in my stomach. After the call, I spotted my mind playing back the conversation several times, imagining us on the phone, how he was sitting and feeling and what he thought of me. In the past, I've noticed patterns of avoidance when helping others in grief. It's only by filling out the record that the habitual tendencies can be seen so clearly.

**Reflection:
Habitual Tendencies in Difficult Communications**

If you're doing the mini-course, simply note in your journal what habitual tendencies you have discovered in the more difficult communications you deal with. Nobody is perfect at communication—we're all human. Everyone has his or her different challenges. Keep this self-compassionate attitude in mind as you reflect on your imperfect communication this week.

Exploring Communication

The word communication comes from the Latin *communicare*, meaning to join, unite, or literally to make common. But how often is communication unifying?

Human beings are social animals, and the heart of socializing lies in effective communication. By communicating well with others, you are able to resolve your differences, build trust, share ideas, and find solutions. Although communication seems simple, poor communication can lead to misunderstanding and swiftly to disagreements, conflict, and stress. Mindfulness offers a way of improving communication so you are better able to connect with your family, friends, and colleagues.

Think about all the communications that you've had today so far. You may have sent text messages, e-mails, or tweets. You may have had a phone conversation or left a voicemail. And of course, you may have had a face-to-face conversation with one or several people already. But communication is not just about sharing ideas. Communication is about sharing emotions. And you can't share emotions that you are not tuned in to. Mindfulness helps you get in touch with both your emotions and those of the other person. This is a vital part of effective communication with others. In this way, you are even able to communicate negative issues in a way that resolves rather than fires up conflict.

Before learning mindfulness, I almost never communicated my emotions to others. My cultural upbringing discouraged the sharing of emotions. After learning mindfulness, in which I got more in touch with my feelings, I began to share my emotions in trusted groups. Now I'm more capable of both listening to others sharing their feelings and sharing my own. It's an aspect of my personality I'm developing, and mindfulness together with journaling my emotions has been a helpful part of that journey.

For example, on one occasion I was given a leadership role in a school and then, several months later, was told that I'd have to step down. No good reason or warning was given. I was understandably angry with the manager and could feel the frustration building up in my body. I managed the situation mindfully by practicing a mindful pause and then writing down all my feelings in a journal that evening. This helped me gather my thoughts and clarify my feelings. The next day I felt comfortable enough to share my experience with close colleagues. They told me about other people who had been treated in the same way by the same manager. I immediately realized the manager was just unskillful in the way he treated staff and felt instantly less stressed—it wasn't all my fault!

Lack of effective communication leads to stress in the following ways:

- Your emotions can fester. Those pent-up emotions can cause you stress.
- You can't put the issue into perspective. In my example, I was able to let go of the stress once I realized the manager had an issue with people management. Problems can seem huge until you share them—then you can realize things aren't quite so bad.
- You get stuck in ruminative thinking. Ever notice how problems can go around and around in your head, generating unnecessary stress? By simply talking it through with someone, you can find an effective solution or at least feel better. A problem shared is indeed a problem halved.

DISCOVER: MINDFUL COMMUNICATION

Mindful communication is a way of communicating more meaningfully in your personal and professional life. Through mindful communication you really tune in to both the content and the emotions of the speaker. Simultaneously, you can consciously respond to your own emotions rather than automatically reacting to them.

The Problem with Autopilot

One of the key challenges in effective communication is autopilot. Autopilot, as you recall from Chapter 4, is living habitually rather than consciously. And although habits can be positive, they can prevent you from making choices and seeing the miracle of life unfolding in front of your eyes—it's like a form of sleepwalking.

When you relate to others automatically, you create conditions for a reactive way of communicating. If the other person says something disagreeable to you, you may react by lashing out with anger, sinking into sadness, or just walking away. Without mindfulness, it just happens—you have no choice.

With mindfulness, you can take the following three steps instead, depicted in the diagram below.

1. **Notice** that your communication is currently happening automatically. You are sitting in the same posture, with the same attitude, jumping to the same conclusions, and feeling the same way as you have many times before.
2. **Connect** with your senses. Look at the person for the first time, practice listening deeply, notice your bodily sensations and reactions. This brings you into the present moment and gives access to all the information you need, both words and emotions, so you can choose to respond more wisely.
3. Make a **choice and act**. Decide how you will respond in this communication. Try choosing something different from your normal, habitual reaction. If it feels uncomfortable, it's a good sign that you've stepped out of habitual mode.

Hiroto had another challenge: his mother. Hiroto's mom always seemed to focus on the negative, and so Hiroto just avoided her. The next time the phone rang and his mother was on the line, Hiroto began arguing back in his habitual way. But then he noticed that he was on autopilot. He connected with his breathing and his body sitting on the bed and then chose to listen mindfully rather than mechanically. It wasn't easy. He felt wave after wave of emotions as his mother spoke. But at the end of an hour's talk, his mother stopped and asked Hiroto how he was. That was different! She had pretty

Notice the habitual, automatic, mindless, choiceless communication

Connect with your senses to bring you into the present

Make a different choice in your communication and take that action much never asked that before. Somehow by being mindful, Hiroto felt his mother had gained permission to step out of her mindless ways too. Over the coming months, he looked forward to the challenge of being mindful with his mother as their relationship began to bloom.

Mindful Listening

> "I've been married for 21 years but now see I've been living automatically for most of that time. Thinking about what I'm grateful for in the relationship has woken me from sleepwalking through my life. After that, to say 'I love you' and really mean it warms my heart."

Have you ever had the experience of speaking to someone and discovered the person hasn't been listening? He asks a question that you just answered or starts arguing rather than appreciating the difficult day that you've been suffering.

Listening itself is almost effortless. The challenge is setting aside all the other thoughts, desires, and emotions that may form a barrier to your listening. Mindful listening is about that process of letting go.

There are several benefits of mindful listening:

- **You build trust.** The speaker will feel like she is being heard, which of course is what she wants if she's speaking! If the speaker feels she is being heard, she's more likely to find a deeper connection. Trust will naturally arise.
- **Conflicts recede**. When you are better able to understand the other person, you're less likely to get into conflict in the first place. In this way, the speaker won't get frustrated.
- **You can soothe emotions** in the speaker. If the speaker is emotionally charged, offering mindful listening will make her feel like the emotion and the problem is being shared, and this helps to reduce the emotion's intensity. In such a case, by listening you are offering an act of kindness. From this place, you are in a position to create a mental space in which a solution or different way of thinking can arise in the speaker or yourself.

Mindful listening in conversation is like a meditation. When you're practicing mindful listening in meditation, the idea is to be open and listen to the sounds, and each time your mind wanders to other thoughts, you gently and kindly bring your attention back, again and again. When listening to the sounds, you avoid being judgmental. Instead you listen with genuine curiosity, care, and acceptance, as best you can.

EXERCISE: Listening Mindfully

Try this in your next conversation:

1. **Prepare** for the communication. Practice a short mindful pause or at least take a few breaths or connect with one of your senses.
2. **Set aside judgment of the person.** If you're holding your own judgment while the other person is speaking, you're not listening to the person—you're listening to your judgment. If you can't do this, try labeling the thought "judgment" and imagine putting the judgment in a box or on a cloud and letting it float away for the time being. You don't have to agree with everything the person says, but you don't have to judge him as a person either.
3. Give the speaker your full and undivided **attention.** Listen to each sentence he says. Notice both the words and the tone of voice.
4. You will probably and quite naturally **nod or say "uh-huh"** as the person speaks. This is more natural than just staring at him without acknowledging what he says and both makes the speaker feel more comfortable and reassures him that you're listening and not spaced out!
5. **Be curious and show curiosity.** Look interested. Adopt open, interested body language. Look at the speaker and use appropriate facial expressions. Ask questions to help clarify the person's point and to show your curiosity.

Have you ever noticed people sometimes pretend to listen? You can tell from their facial expression and body language that they're not listening. They're just waiting to jump in and make their point. They're just listening to their own ideas. If they listened carefully, the conversation would be far more productive. Ensure you don't get caught in that habit too. Make sure you're not just acting as if you're listening, but actually listening.

Interruptions are another issue in conversations. Do you find yourself interrupting the speaker? If you find yourself interrupting with statements like "Oh, yes, the same thing happened to me when . . . ," your attention is on your own thoughts rather than the speaker. Conversations are not about looking for chances to speak, but begin with simply understanding what the speaker is sharing. When I catch myself interrupting someone, I know it's time to step back and practice mindful listening more diligently.

Reflection

1. Think back to a time when you communicated well with someone. When was it, who were you with, what was your state of mind, and what were you talking about? How did it feel to communicate effectively? How mindful were you in that communication? Consider how you can apply your experience to future communications.

2. Now consider a difficult communication that you handled well. How did you manage this? What was the quality of your listening like? How can you apply this to future difficult communications?

Jot your thoughts down in your journal if you like.

BEYOND WORDS: NONVERBAL COMMUNICATION

When you talk about something important to you, nonverbal communication conveys more than your actual words. Nonverbal communication includes body language, facial expression, tone of voice, eye contact, and gestures. And to a more subtle extent, even breathing and muscle tension can have an effect. Your emotions are expressed far more nonverbally than from what you actually say.

By understanding nonverbal communication, you can express yourself and comprehend the other person more effectively. This can be particularly helpful to resolve conflict in difficult conversations. I like to think of this as listening with your eyes and not just your ears.

Use open body language by uncrossing your arms and looking the other person in the eye when she speaks.

Enhancing How You Interpret Nonverbal Communication

A great way to help develop your skills in learning nonverbal communication is to watch others. I love to sit in cafés and people-watch, trying to guess the emotional state and relationship between people by looking at nonverbal communication. When you can't hear what they're saying, you start to learn more about nonverbal communication. Even watching television without the sound on can teach you the power of body language. It's great practice.

A couple of things to remember, though:

1. **People of different cultures, ages, and genders use different body language, so don't read too deeply into each signal.** For example, while good eye contact is almost the norm in the West, it's seen as disrespectful in other

areas, including some Asian and African cultures. The less eye contact these groups have, the more respect they show.

2. **And consider a group of body language signals as a whole rather than just one.** For example, if someone happens to have her arms crossed for a while, it doesn't mean she's definitely afraid or feeling defensive—maybe she's just feeling a bit cold without her jacket. But if she also avoids eye contact, looks away a lot, and is a bit jumpy, it might be safer to conclude she's worried about something.

Research Corner:
How Your Posture Can Transform Your Life

Social psychologist Amy Cuddy wondered: Can deliberately adopting a confident posture for 2 minutes affect one's level of stress?

She took two random groups of people. One group had to adopt an open body pose, which normally signifies high confidence and power—for example, sitting back with chest open and arms behind the head. The other group adopted a closed body posture with arms and legs folded, which implied low confidence.

After 2 minutes of holding the high-confidence pose, participants' saliva was tested. The results of the short test were amazing. The open body pose group had lowered their stress hormone cortisol by about 25%! The closed body pose participants ended up with 10% higher levels of cortisol.

In another study by Cuddy, adopting the high-confidence pose for 2 minutes before an interview greatly increased the chance of being hired. It was even more important than what the interviewee actually said or what qualifications the applicant had. The main reason: the pose made people have greater *presence.*

So try this. Next time you're faced with a stressful situation like being interviewed, making a presentation, teaching a class, or seeing your doctor, take 2 minutes to mindfully open your posture. Go to the bathroom or to your office or into the elevator and really open up your body. Just 2 minutes. Stand up and make a big star sign with your body (just spread your arms and legs far apart), and do it mindfully. Feel your breathing, your body sensations, your emotions. Your stress levels will drop and your sense of confidence will rise—the science backs it up. For an interview or presentation, those 2 minutes could change the direction your life.

Developing Your Own Nonverbal Communication

The basic skill in nonverbal communication is to match your words to your body language. If you're speaking about something you're excited about, you need to be smiling, have a slightly faster rate of speaking and higher tone of voice and appropriate gestures with your arms, for example. If your words don't match your nonverbal communication, the listener won't believe you.

TIP One excellent way to use body language is when you're feeling anxious about a meeting, like a date. If you stand upright, smile and maintain eye contact, and speak a bit more slowly, even though you feel scared, your emotions may start to ease. This is a clever way to use your body to ease your emotions.

Stress and Mindful Communication

As you've already read, a bit of pressure is fine and part of life. But constant or high levels of stress take a toll on your relationships. This is because your brain's high-level functioning gets shut down by the fight-or-flight response and you're much more likely to react in a way that you later regret—an experience most people have had. Mindful communication can help you both prevent stress from rising too high and discover ways to respond quickly to that stress so it doesn't cause further difficulties in your relationships.

When you're in the middle of a heated conversation with your boss, you can't stop for 10 minutes of meditation! So how can you help to relieve your stress so the communication doesn't get out of control? Here are a few suggestions.

PRACTICE: Dealing with Stress during a Conversation

These techniques can be put into play whenever you feel stressed during a conversation. The more you practice with them, the more easily you'll be able to apply them when needed.

1. **Recognize** that your stress level is rising. Look out for your stress signals such as tension in your shoulders, increased heart rate, a constant need to interrupt the speaker, or a tightening in your chest, for example. Or you may close down and feel like running away, looking downward, or freezing.

2. **Take a breath.** Feel one full in- and out-breath, even while the person is speaking. Switch your attention for a few seconds into the physical sensation of your breathing. Breathe in and out through your nose so that you don't look like you're sighing in frustration.

3. **Connect with a sense.** Choose whatever works for you. For me, I like the physical sensation of my feet on the floor or my body on the chair. You may prefer noticing what the speaker looks like with curiosity, listening to all the sounds around you as well as what the speaker is saying.

4. **Look for the middle ground.** If you're willing to compromise, you may find a place where it's not ideal for you or the person, but at least you do find a resolution to the issue. Not being willing to compromise at all will often just lead to more stressful communication, and isn't the most effective way to be with others. You both have needs and desires.

5. **See the funny side.** I know this can be much more difficult in the heat of a stressful conversation, but humor can be a great way to dissipate the tension. If you can look at things from a bigger picture, you may be able to see the light-hearted aspects of the situation.

(TIP) If you find yourself getting stressed in certain relationships, personal or professional, and just can't seem to stop, rather than trying harder and harder to manage your stress, just watch. Just be as mindful as you can of the conversation and the stress, without trying to stop any emotions or frustrations. Notice your body, the sentences that pour out of your mouth, and the tension that rises. And if you forget to be mindful, be aware of that too! Observing your own behavior with mindfulness and compassion sets the stage for transformation by itself.

MINDFUL COMMUNICATION AND EMOTIONS

Communication is usually motivated by emotions, and difficult communications are often charged with those emotions. So the quality of the communication depends on an awareness of both your emotions and the emotions of the other person. For example, if you're feeling anxious but don't know it, you may find yourself shouting at your partner about a small issue rather than talking about the real cause of your stress.

If you lack awareness of how you're feeling, you won't be able to share your emotions and needs with others. And if you aren't aware of the other person's feelings, you won't be able to understand or help him either. This lack of awareness leads to frustration in both parties, as needs are left unfulfilled.

Mindfulness of emotions is a vital life skill. You may be frightened of strong emotions like sadness or anger, but when you ignore, suppress, or fight the emotions, they become a bigger problem. Mindfulness of emotions helps you become aware of emotions with acceptance, so you can respond to the feeling by either just staying with the sensation or deciding to communicate the emotion in an appropriate way. Simply venting anger is a reaction to the feeling of anger and not often appropriate or helpful; learning to be with the emotion and expressing it well is far more satisfying and effective.

EXERCISE: Assessing Your Emotional Awareness

Answer the following questions to assess your general emotional awareness. Jot your thoughts down in your journal if that helps:

- Do you ever feel emotions as a physical sensation?
- Do you ever use emotions or gut feelings to guide your decisions?
- Do you pay attention to your constantly changing inner emotional landscape rather than noticing only one or two emotions in the day?
- Are you comfortable with all your feelings and willing to share your emotions with others?
- Are you sensitive to other people's emotions by putting yourself in their shoes?

The more questions you answered with a no, the less you are currently mindful of your emotions. You can boost your mindful awareness of emotions and therefore improve your communication by:

- Practicing mindfulness of emotions, which is part of the **expanding awareness meditation** in Chapter 8.
- **Labeling your emotions** in your mind as you experience them, whether they are pleasant or not.
- **Asking yourself,** "How am I feeling? Where do I feel this emotion in my body?" several times a day.
- **Sharing your emotions** with a trusted friend.
- **Keeping a journal** and writing down your reflections and emotions from the day or after a difficult communication.

EXERCISE: Mindful Speaking and Listening

Here's an exercise that you can do with someone else—your partner, a friend, or anyone. The exercise takes about 5 minutes.

1. Begin by **asking your partner to talk** to you about any topic she wishes for 5 minutes. Use a timer.
2. **Listen mindfully without interrupting.** You can do this listening by using the techniques taught on page 190.
3. Remember to **use your nonverbal communication skills,** including looking the person in the eyes, acknowledging that you're listening to him, and also noticing any thoughts and feelings that may be arising for you and setting them aside for the time being.
4. You can just **think of it like a meditation** rather than your normal way of listening. This way of listening will help you go from the normal automatic pilot or habitual way of listening to this more mindful form of listening.
5. When the time is up, you can **switch roles.** This time you're doing the speaking and the other person can practice mindful listening.
6. When you're speaking, you can take your time to speak, noticing what you're saying and listening to your tone of voice. If you feel too self-conscious, let go of this process. But I know for me personally, listening to my tone of voice makes me more mindful and makes me speak more slowly and eloquently.

GOING DEEPER: Practice a mindful pause before and after speaking and before and after listening. And if you want to challenge yourself even further, talk about an issue that's more emotionally charged for you.

Reflection

At the end of the exercise, discuss your findings. What did you discover about yourself and your friend? What did you enjoy? What did you find challenging? Did you find it easier to do the listening part of the process or the speaking? Is that the same experience in your daily life? Specifically focus on the process of speaking and listening mindfully.

Mindful Assertiveness: Beyond Passive and Aggressive

When you're assertive, you're able to express your needs and desires as well as respect the other person, and this leads to more authentic and harmonious communications and relationships. Most people confuse assertiveness with aggressiveness, however. When you're being assertive in your communication, you're being neither aggressive nor passive.

Research Corner: Journaling Is like Medicine

I've offered lots of opportunities to journal in this book. Here's some research that touches on the health benefits of journaling.

University of Texas Psychology Professor and Chair Dr. James Pennebaker is considered the grandfather of journaling research. In his classic study in 1988, 50 students were assigned to journal about either their life's most traumatic experiences, or everyday experiences, for 4 days in a row. Six weeks later, he found those that journaled about their traumatic life experiences had more positive moods, fewer illnesses, improved cellular immune-system function, and fewer visits to the student health center—all compared to those writing about everyday experiences. Confronting traumatic experiences seemed to be physically beneficial.

In another study called "Effects of Writing about Stressful Experiences on Symptom Reduction in Patients with Asthma or Rheumatoid Arthritis," published in the *Journal of the American Medical Association* in 1999, 112 patients with asthma or rheumatoid arthritis participated. A group of them were asked to journal for about 20 minutes a day for 3 consecutive days about the *most traumatic event of their lives*. So just 1 hour in total. Four months later, almost 50% of the group journaling about their stressful event showed a clinically significant improvement in their condition! The report stated that if a medicine were found to have the same effects, its use would be widespread within a short time.

I think by expressing emotions on paper, the participants became more mindful of their suppressed feelings and this lowered their levels of stress, boosting their immune system and making them healthier. It's an easy and inexpensive way to manage your stress in a relatively short time. Give it a go sometime!

A mindfully assertive person communicates her needs
with clarity and sensitivity. An aggressive person
demands her needs without care.

I use the term mindful assertiveness to emphasize that it's not just about asserting your own rights but about being sensitive to the needs of others as well. Mindful assertiveness is about practicing assertiveness in the backdrop of a compassionate mindful awareness of your own mind-set and that of the other person.

OVERCOMING PASSIVE COMMUNICATION

If you're passive in your communication, you're more likely to agree to the wishes of others even though it undermines your needs. If you have a strong desire to be liked by others, you'll have a tendency to be passive.

My own personality leans toward being passive, even though I am quite an extrovert. I didn't think that meditation would help me be more assertive. But actually, through meditation I'm much better able to handle emotions like anxiety. When I do have to complain or stand up for myself, I use it as an opportunity to practice mindfulness, rather than avoiding the discomfort and acting passively. I usually enjoy that challenge now.

Passive people are often considered kind and friendly, just like mindfully assertive people. But they have trouble being kind and friendly to themselves. They don't see themselves as of equal importance to other people. If this sounds like you, combining mindfulness with assertiveness skills could help lower your stress.

For example, if your sister asked you to pick up some bread from the store, a passive response might be "I'm busy looking after the children and need to take Jonny for his piano lesson and promised Michael I'd cook dinner, but I'll squeeze it in just before that." A more assertive response might be "No, I don't have time for that today. I'm really busy. Sorry I can't help you this time."

Saying yes to someone might mean saying no
to something else. Think before you agree to someone
else's request.

Assertiveness training has traditionally said to avoid apologizing. But mindful assertiveness is about being friendly and kind as well as firm. The idea is to try to create a win–win situation so both parties are at least a little bit satisfied.

PRACTICE: Mindfully Responding to Requests

The next time you get a request to do something, become aware of how you're feeling. If you find yourself automatically saying yes again, just notice. Practice a mindful pause after the conversation. Then consider your own needs just as much as the other person's needs. If you feel you're probably being too kind to the other person but not kind to yourself at all, call the person back and politely say you can't fulfill the request. When you practice this periodically, you become more comfortably assertive.

REDUCING AGGRESSIVE COMMUNICATION

When you respond aggressively in your communication, you're saying you see your desires, needs, and rights as greater than those of others. Aggressive responding includes telling rather than asking, rushing the other person unnecessarily, not taking feelings into account—even ignoring is a form of aggression.

An aggressive form of communication lacks compassion. An aggressive person is not seeing the situation from the other person's perspective, only his own. If you make an aggressive communication, you're more likely to provoke either a passive or an aggressive response. If the other person responds aggressively, you're unlikely to get your needs or desires met. And if the other person responds passively, you would have made that person feel low or more stressed rather than strengthening the relationship.

Tales of Wisdom: The Starfish Story

Once upon a time a man was walking along a beach when he noticed a boy in the distance hurriedly throwing something into the sea. He approached the boy and said, "Hey, what are you up to?"

"I'm throwing starfish back into the ocean. The tide is going out, and if I don't throw them back in, they'll die," replied the boy.

The man laughed. "Look along the coastline. There's thousands of starfish. You can't possibly make a difference!"

The boy listened patiently. Then he looked down, picked up another starfish, and gently threw it back into the ocean. He smiled back at the man and said, "I made a difference to that one."

What does the story mean to you? To me, it reminds me that every small act of kindness *does* make a difference.

PRACTICE: Mindfully Noticing Others' Reactions
to You

Notice other people's reactions when you communicate with them. Notice their facial expression, body language, and tone of voice. If people tend to react with defensiveness or aggression, perhaps you're being too aggressive in your communication. Just observe to begin with before judging yourself or making any changes. Do this whenever you think of it during an interaction to become more mindfully aware of the effect you might be having on others. Avoid the temptation to change at first— just watch to begin with. Your change will happen naturally if you watch people's reactions nonjudgmentally.

BEING MINDFULLY ASSERTIVE

To be mindfully assertive means to take a balanced view of your own needs as well as the needs of the other person. You express your needs, but you also listen to the needs of others and seek to find an amicable solution.

These are the kinds of behaviors that are part of mindful assertiveness:

- Mindfully listening to others and letting go of your judgment while they speak.
- Both accepting your responsibilities and being willing to delegate to others.
- Being aware of your own emotions and avoiding reacting to them habitually; instead you respond to them with conscious awareness of making a choice.
- Being willing to apologize when you're wrong.
- Being grateful for what others are doing for you and sharing your appreciation with others.
- Balancing a kindness to yourself with a kindness toward others.
- Forgiving yourself when you're too passive or aggressive and making small changes to be a bit more assertive next time.

Here are two mindful techniques to be more assertive in your communication.

Traffic Light Communication

Author Susan Chapman specializes in mindful communication. She likes to use the model of traffic lights when teaching mindful communication skills.

Red light represents being closed down and defensive. Your husband turns up an hour late at the restaurant and doesn't even apologize. An argument ensues. Your focus turns to your own needs rather than anyone else. You don't care about the relationship, only that he's rude and you're starving. You can be in a red light communication zone for minutes, hours, days, years, or even a lifetime.

Yellow light is in between. Your husband is late for dinner, but you're not totally overwhelmed by your emotions. There's an opportunity to make a choice. You could go down the red route and turn passive or aggressive. But you have an option. With a dash of mindful awareness and the possibility of responding differently to the situation, you make matters better. You soothe your emotions by connecting with your senses and enjoying the restaurant's aromas. You give him a kiss and order starters. Lateness can be discussed afterward. You're moving toward green light instead of red.

Green light is openness. With openness you can access compassion, curiosity, and acceptance. This is the state of mindfulness. The needs of others are just as valuable as your own. You can love, care, and both feel the pain of others and a desire to relieve that pain. You react with concern to your husband's late arrival and are pleased to see he has arrived safe and well. Before long, there's laughter, engaging conversation, and a plate of pasta.

By being mindful of your traffic light signal, you can make better choices in your communication. Take close care about what you do and say in red, exercise your ability to make the right choice when in yellow, and enjoy deepening your communication when green.

PRACTICE: **Find the Truth**

This is a great technique you can practice using any time someone is being aggressive toward you. Your response is then neither aggressive nor passive. Simply look for an element of truth in the person's statement and agree with that, even if it's a bit critical.

Here's how:

1. **Listen** to what the person says.
2. **Notice** any strong emotions arising in your body and feel them with your breathing.

3. In a calm way, make your statement, **highlighting the truth.**
4. **Listen mindfully again,** without judging the person as "bad," as this evokes more conflict and stress. Instead, listen and seek the element of truth.
5. Again, use mindfulness to accept and step back from your thoughts and **repeat** any true element.

For example:

OTHER: You haven't cooked dinner yet! You're so lazy! (*aggressive tone*)

YOU: Yes, I haven't cooked dinner yet. (*calm response*)

OTHER: I've been working so hard. I'm tired and hungry. What's wrong with you?! (*still aggressive*)

YOU: Yes, I know you're hungry and tired and have been working hard. I've been busy with the children, actually. I plan to make dinner soon. (*Identifies truth again. Uses breath to stay calm.*)

OTHER: Oh, I see. I'll look after them. (*much calmer response*)

PRACTICE: Empathic Assertion

This is a conscious way of acknowledging how the other person feels before you express your need. In this way you show empathy. Simply start your statement with how the other person sees the situation.

For example, here someone starts with acknowledging the parking attendant:

"I understand you say you don't normally offer refunds for parking tickets."

Then follow this with your need:

"However, in this case, I paid for my parking, so I would like a refund, please."

Acknowledging what the other person says can make him less defensive and make a resolution more likely. This takes practice and mindfulness, however, since emotions are often high. Practice in less heated interactions at first and then work your way up to the most tense situations.

Enacting Communication Styles: Learning through Movement

In my workshops, I like to get people to act out different poses to experience different communication styles: passive, aggressive, and mindful communication. This way of exploring emotions is particularly effective if you learn through activity and movement rather than just reading.

I describe three different role-play scenarios below. Try them out with your partner or a friend when you can.

EXERCISE: Communicating Passively

In this exercise, you are going to enact a passive form of communication using physical role play rather than actually exchanging words.

1. Begin by facing your partner, about 6 feet apart. Center yourself with a few breaths and tune in to your emotional state.
2. Ask the other person to raise his arms parallel to the floor and come toward you.
3. As he gets close to pushing you, lie down on the floor in a passive way, giving in.
4. The other person simply walks around you as you lie there.

Reflection

Write down your thoughts in your journal if you like.

What did you feel during this interaction? What were your thoughts? Did this feel like a familiar form of communication, or was it alien to you? How would you have preferred to respond rather than lying down?

EXERCISE: Communicating Aggressively

This time, you are going to enact an aggressive form of communication using physical role play rather than actually exchanging words.

1. Begin by facing your partner, about 6 feet apart.

2. Ask your partner to raise her arms parallel to the floor while you do the same.
3. Move toward each other and push against each other, without knocking anyone over!
4. Continue to push each other. The harder your partner pushes, the harder you need to push back.

Reflection

How did you feel during this exercise? How did it compare to your emotions in the first scenario? What thoughts arose for you this time? Some people feel more empowered in this aggressive form of communication compared to the passive example earlier. Others feel uncomfortable, as if it's unnatural.

EXERCISE: ## Communicating with Mindful Assertiveness

In this final exercise, you are going to model a mindfully assertive form of communication using physical role play. Again, this is done in silence. This time, hold a very slight smile on your face too—to remind you to be playful in the interaction.

1. Raise your arms in front of you, parallel to the floor, and have your partner do the same.
2. As your partner moves toward you, move toward her too, looking her in the eye.
3. As she moves toward you, take hold of her wrists and use their force to gently direct their energy to one side rather than toward you.
4. Use the force in your partner's arms to move in almost a dance, continuing to flow with each other. Take a firm stand and neither run away nor exert full control. Play with the forces your partner exerts and put a little bit of force in yourself to redirect the energy.

5. Stay aware, moment by moment. Acknowledge the other person's point of view through her physical movement and express your point of view by physically guiding her arms in the way you wish. You don't know where you'll be moving next, and you're open to that, trusting yourself in each moment to make a choice as to which direction to move in.

I personally really enjoy this exercise. You get to experience physically what it's like to allow the physical force that someone exerts on you without too

> "I've always had a fiery personality. It led to the breakdown of a relationship that I really valued—I was distraught. Mindfulness helped me see my fear underneath the anger and gave me the skills to soothe that anxiety with my breath and self-kindness. I'm not in a new relationship, but I'm far more at peace with myself."

Thich Nhat Hanh on Communication

Nobel Peace Prize nominee and the second-most-famous Buddhist monk after the Dalai Lama is Zen Buddhist mindfulness teacher Thich Nhat Hanh. Here is a summary of his key advice on what he calls mindful or compassionate communication.

The essence of communication is deep listening and loving speech.

Deep listening—Listen with compassion to relieve the suffering of the other person. Even if the other person is mistaken in his interpretation of a situation, just listen deeply. Correct his interpretation when you think he'd be ready to listen—but not now. For now, don't interrupt or argue; just listen with your heart. An hour of this can bring about healing and transformation in the other person.

Loving speech—There is a saying in Vietnamese that "It doesn't cost anything to have loving speech." When dealing with a difficult conversation, use loving speech. And ask for help. For example: "'Darling, I am suffering, and I want you to know it. Darling, I am doing my best; I'm trying not to blame anyone else, including you. Since we are so close to each other, since we have made a commitment to each other, I feel that I need your support and your help to get out of this state of suffering, of anger."

The practice of mindfulness meditation and living mindfully in everything you do will help you listen deeply and speak lovingly.

much effort. It's a bit like a freestyle dancing where you play off each other's movement. When you're dancing, it's doesn't feel like effort—it's fun. You don't know what will happen next. One moment you're going around in a circle, and the next minute your partner is doing spins and you're both laughing. It's a great metaphor for meeting difficult conversations in a different way rather than just hiding, running away, or fighting back.

GOING DEEPER: If you enjoyed the role plays, try some more! One involves curling yourself into a ball when the other person comes toward you. Yet another involves running away as the other person comes toward you. Try them out if you have time, and make up one of your own. There are so many different ways we all react in communication, both one to one and in a group. Also try to apply the advice of Thich Nhat Hanh whenever you can, summarized in the box on page 205.

Reflection

What feelings arose for you as you did this exercise? What thoughts arose in your mind? Did you enjoy this process, or did you find it difficult? Did the movement turn into a form of dance, or did you still feel some sort of fight or resistance with your partner?

PRACTICE: Mindful Yoga

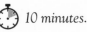 10 minutes.

30 minutes.

Audio tracks 9 and 10.

Practice the mini or full mindful yoga sequence in Chapter 13.

PRACTICE: Expanding Awareness
Mindfulness Meditation

 10 minutes.

30 minutes.

Audio tracks 15 and 16.

This week the expanding awareness meditation practice is just the same as you did last week. Remember to choose either the mini or full version. Try it now by finding a comfortable yet upright posture and using the guided audio.

GOING DEEPER: RESPONDING TO YOUR STRESS MEDITATION. At the end of the meditation, try the following exercise.

 5–10 minutes.

Audio track 17.

1. Bring to mind a **current challenge** in your life that is the cause of some stress. A situation that you're willing to work with at the moment. Not your biggest challenge but not so small that it causes no stress at all. A 3 on a scale of 1–10 is a good guide.
2. **Bring the situation vividly to mind.** Imagine being in the situation and all the difficulties associated with it.
3. Notice whether you can **feel the stress in your body.** Physical tension, faster heart rate, a little bit of sweating, butterflies in your stomach, tightness in the back or shoulders or jaw, perhaps. Look out for your stress signals.
4. **Tune in to your emotions.** Notice how you feel. Label that emotion if you can, and be aware of where you feel the emotion, exactly, in your body. Just try to spot it as best you can. The more precisely you can locate the emotion and the more you notice about the sensation, the better. With time and experience, you'll keep getting better at this.
5. **Bring mindful attitudes to the emotion.** These include curiosity, friendliness, and acceptance.
6. **Try placing your hand** on the location of the sensation—a friendly

hand representing kindness. Do it the way you would place your hand on the injured knee of a child, with care and affection.

7. **Feel the sensation together with your breathing.** This can promote a present-moment awareness and mindful attitudes to your experience.

8. When you're ready, bring this meditation to a close.

Reflection

What effect did the responding to your stress meditation have on you? Write down your experience and reflections.

This is an important and challenging meditation, teaching you the skills to be with stress and its emotions without reacting to them but instead learning to be with those difficult sensations.

Preparing for a Day of Mindfulness

At some point this week, the MBSR program includes a full day of mindfulness practice. This will be detailed in the next chapter. If you're doing the mini-program, you don't have to do this. If you're doing the full program and are seeking the maximum benefits from mindfulness, look at your schedule and see how you could make time for a day of mindfulness. At this point all you need to do is make time for a day of mindfulness in which you don't have any other responsibilities.

The benefits of a day of mindfulness are:

- An opportunity to **deepen** your experience of mindful awareness as you move from one mindfulness practice to another.
- A chance to **discover** how your body and mind respond to an extended period of mindfulness practice.
- The **time** to train your mind in mindfulness for an extended period of time without going back into your normal habits.

I remember on the last day of mindfulness that I ran for teacher training, one lady had tears rolling down her cheeks at the end. She explained in an animated way that the experience of spending a day just being mindful and resting was exactly what she needed. Her father had died a couple of years before, and she'd blocked herself from the grief. She thought she wouldn't be able to handle it. The day gave her the space to stop avoiding the feelings and the courage to allow them to come through slowly. It was totally unexpected. A few months later she said that day was a major breakthrough in her life and she now felt happier and more confident.

Reflection: How Are the Home Experiments Going?

1. How have the expanding awareness meditation and body scan or mindful yoga home experiments been going? What went well? What did you struggle with?

2. If you didn't practice on certain days, what thoughts did you have? What got in the way?

Meditation and Mindful Stretching FAQs

Q: **I've really taken to the yoga, but the body scan and expanding aware-ness meditation don't work for me. Can I stop them?**

A: All these meditations work in subtle ways in their own time. Just because you don't immediately feel the benefits doesn't mean they're not working. So as you made a commitment at the beginning of the course to stick it out for the 8 weeks, give it a shot. It's just 3 more weeks! And then you can make your decision.

Q: **I was hoping my mind chatter would calm down after all this medita-tion, but it hasn't really stopped. Am I doing something wrong?**

A: Mind chatter is here to stay, I'm afraid. Sometimes it calms down and sometimes it increases, like when you're under stress. The great thing about mindfulness is that you can carry on being mindful despite the mind chatter. You can acknowledge the mind chatting away and come back to focusing on your breathing or your partner's concerns or the tree by the road. Think of your mind chatter like the weather outside—it's almost always changing. Give up all hope to silence the chatter and give full attention as best you can to being mindful; that's the less stressful approach. You don't need to make mind chatter another problem to deal with. *Use mind chatter as a stepping stone into mindful awareness.*

Q: I think I've overstretched myself in the yoga. I'm so stupid. I'm limping around when I try to walk. What should I do?

A: You're not stupid for doing that. What sort of thought is "I'm so stupid"? It's a self-judgment. Notice your mind patterns here. You've judged yourself for making a mistake as a beginner in yoga. Interesting, isn't it? See if you can spot that happening at other times in your daily life. That's what mindfulness is about!

Q: I prefer to do the meditations without the audio. Is that okay?

A: Yes, that's fine. You can choose from tracks 20 to 23, which is just silence with bells to let you know when it's time to stop.

Q: Why do we do mindfulness of thoughts? The whole reason I'm doing this is to stop paying attention to negative thoughts; if I pay attention to those thoughts, I know where I'll end up, and it's not a good place.

> It's very common for beginners to go too far. I've made this mistake too! You're discovering your body's current limits and gone past your edge; it's part of the discovery process in yoga. Have a break, and when you feel better, restart the practice and go easy on the stretches. Mindful yoga is a mindfulness exercise more than a physical exercise.

A: First of all, all the exercises are your choice. If you feel they are not right for you, remember you can stop them. The reason for practicing mindfulness of thoughts is not to go down your usual habitual thinking paths but to look at them as if you're separate from them— like you see clouds in the sky. You can't stop clouds from coming into the sky. You also can't stop thoughts from coming into your mind; it's what thoughts do.

EXERCISE: Paper Thought Clouds

If you're having trouble stepping back from you thoughts, this exercise is a fun one to try. Take some paper and cut it into the shape of clouds. Write some of your common thoughts on the clouds. Then pass them in front of your eyes so they come into vision from your left and go out of sight on your right while you look straight ahead. There's no need to dwell further about each thought cloud. See if you can see each thought in the same way—as on another cloud. Do this several times, until the thoughts seem to have almost the same emotionally uncharged effect. Then throw the clouds in the trash or burn them—this can enhance the feeling of letting the thoughts go. Note any insights you had about this exercise in your journal, if you wish.

Home Experiments: Week 6

This week's main home experiment alternates between expanding awareness meditation and either the body scan or a mindful yoga sequence of your choice. You can choose whatever you feel is right for you each day. Remember to use the table to find out what you need to be practicing this week and keep recording your findings in your journal.

Mindful Booster

This week's mindful booster is to have one mindful communication per day. It could be with someone close to you, or even a brief few minutes with a colleague at work, or at the local store. Remember to stop, look, listen, and avoid interrupting. Keep an open body language and be curious. Notice tone of voice and the other person's body language. Your discoveries could have a big impact on understanding yourself and your relationships, so jot your observations down and take a few moments to reflect on your findings about yourself.

Mindful Pause

If you're doing the full course, practice one of your mindful pauses after a stressful experience. Use this as an opportunity to respond to your experience of stress rather than reacting, if you can. And if you do find yourself reacting automatically to your stress, notice that nonjudgmentally too. Write down your findings.

Week 6

Day	Mini-Course	Full Course
1	Mini-expanding awareness meditation Mindful booster: mindful communication	Full expanding awareness meditation Mindful pause × 3 Mindful booster: mindful communication
2	Mini-body scan or mini-yoga Mindful booster: self-compassion	Full body scan or full yoga Mindful pause × 3 Mindful booster: mindful communication
3	Mini-expanding awareness meditation Mindful booster: mindful communication	Full expanding awareness meditation Mindful pause × 3 Mindful booster: mindful communication
4	Mini-body scan or mini-yoga Mindful booster: mindful communication	Full body scan or full yoga Mindful pause × 3 Mindful booster: mindful communication
5	Mini-expanding awareness meditation Mindful booster: mindful communication	Full expanding awareness meditation Mindful pause × 3 Mindful booster: mindful communication
6	Mini-body scan or mini-yoga Mindful booster: mindful communication	Full body scan or full yoga Mindful pause × 3 Mindful booster: mindful communication

TEN

A Day of Mindfulness

Deepening Your Awareness

Out beyond ideas of wrongdoing and right doing there is a field. I'll meet you there. When the soul lies down in that grass the world is too full to talk about.

—RUMI

INTENTIONS

✦ *To understand the reasons for a day of silent mindfulness practice.*

✦ *To explore the best ways to prepare for the day.*

✦ *To decide what to do on your day of mindfulness.*

✦ *To overcome challenges that typically come up during a day of mindfulness.*

"MY LIFE changed through an insight during a day of mindfulness," said Jayden. His face was beaming. His smile, infectious. He shared his story with us over a cup of tea after a meditation session.

Jayden had first suffered from anxiety when he was studying for exams in high school. In fact, his stomach felt so painful due to the anxiety that he took antacids several times a day to soothe his belly and make the discomfort go away. He felt ashamed of his feelings. Why did this happen only to him? Why did all the other students seem so confident? It wasn't fair. The anxiety continued through college and when he started work for a marketing agency.

One day, strolling home tired after a day at work, Jayden got mugged. He wasn't hurt physically, but he couldn't stop thinking about what could have happened and started to get panic attacks. To make matters worse, a week later, he got mugged again. Life was not good. Focusing at work was becoming impossible, and he was going into a downward spiral. He'd stopped eating properly, couldn't sleep, and felt jumpy and nervous almost all the time.

He shared his recent problems with one of his colleagues. A 10-minute chat turned into an hour-long tearful conversation. Jayden was referred to a therapist by his manager, who turned out to be a keen advocate of mindfulness. After a few months of therapy, his anxiety was getting under control and the mindfulness exercises he had learned seemed to be helping.

Jayden joined a mindfulness class and then a full day of silent mindfulness practice was recommended to him. "In silence!" he thought. He'd never been silent for a whole day; it seemed really crazy. Just 10 minutes or so in the meditations was fine, but a whole day? His therapist encouraged him to try it. Jayden reluctantly agreed to the challenge but began to feel that familiar swirling in the pit of his stomach. The night before, he dived into bed, got into a fetal position, but just couldn't sleep. What had he got himself into? Why was he so scared?

When he arrived for the day of mindfulness, people were having refreshments and chatting outside in the sunshine. Jayden didn't want to talk to anyone; he felt too nervous. He found a place to sit down inside the hall to meditate and did his usual mindful pause to try to settle himself. His thoughts were negative and he had mixed emotions. His neck and shoulders were so tense—he couldn't really feel them.

The first meditation was for half an hour, and Jayden ended it feeling worse rather than better. Next was mindful yoga. That was easier. He began to focus. He initially had thoughts about not being able to stretch, but the stretches were easy. The teacher emphasized keeping eyes closed so no one would be tempted to judge and compare themselves to others and how far or little they can stretch. That was not the point. Keeping eyes closed helped him focus on his own bodily sensations and breathing.

The breakthrough happened for Jayden in one of the meditations he was doing on the meditation cushion. The long periods of meditation and being away from his usual distractions during the day of mindfulness gave Jayden's mind time to calm down. In his more focused state, he was able to see clearly how mindfully accepting anxiety helped. This is the mindful acceptance you learned about in Chapter 8. He felt the familiar anxiety in the pit of his stomach but decided to just really let it be. Rather than mentally trying to push his feeling away, he consciously felt the emotion without too many thoughts distracting him. Like a gentle wave that rises from the ocean, the anxiety rose gracefully and began to fall. He kept watching. Down it went.

The anxiety diminished because Jayden was able to feel the emotion without fearing it. The safe place of the day of mindfulness gave him the time and space to observe without judging—the essence of mindfulness.

The penny had dropped. Before Jayden had been accepting the feeling so that it would go away. But now he was *really* accepting it. He had the genuine attitude of "whatever happens happens." Whether the anxiety was there or not there didn't matter. In fact, he began to *look* for the anxiety rather than get rid of it. It felt like standing up to something scary—like a bully—and that felt empowering.

The day of mindfulness ended well for Jayden, and he went back for more. Regular meditation helps him keep his worries under control and make space for his emotions to pass through his awareness rather than getting stuck within him. Anxiety still comes up for him in the face of stress, but he meets it with a much healthier attitude these days.

Jayden's breakthrough arose in a day of mindfulness practice. But you don't have to do a day's meditation with a group if you don't have access to one. This chapter will show you how to do a day of mindfulness without a teacher. You can then adjust the schedule and content to fit your time and lifestyle. You can even practice with friends or family or try half a day if that's all you have time for.

What Is a Day of Mindfulness?

The purpose of the day of mindfulness is to train your mind to be more present.

A day of mindfulness consists of practicing mindfulness meditation and doing daily activities in a mindful way while being silent. The day starts the moment you wake up and continues until you drift off to sleep.

Being silent, your thinking mind begins to calm and your senses sharpen. Your bodily sensations are more pronounced. And emotions can become heightened—both the difficult and the joyful ones. This is of course a generalization, and different people have different experiences. But I have found everyone is pleasantly surprised by how transformative a day of mindfulness can be.

In your normal, everyday life, there are plenty of distractions—TV, Internet, and cell phones to name a few. Then there are all the responsibilities that you have to fulfill and all the various unexpected problems to deal with. That's a lot to think about. So when you sit to meditate, it's no wonder your mind is still swirling with thoughts and focusing is difficult.

A day of mindfulness is free of responsibilities. You have time simply to be rather than constantly doing. In this time, three benefits arise:

1. Your body and mind have time to de-stress. You're under less pressure from constant doing and so begin to relax—a bit like a vacation without the stressful travel.

2. You discover new insights about how your mind works. You notice patterns like always thinking about the future or feeling guilty when you're not doing something productive. This self-knowledge helps you see why you're feeling stressed and lessens anxiety.

3. Your mind has time to calm down. Normal, everyday stimulation keeps your mind overly active. In this calmer state, you can begin to feel more peaceful and get a sense of clarity.

These benefits are hard to access among your normal, everyday activities because you're just too busy to notice.

I like to practice a day of mindfulness once a month. Often I don't manage this due to other commitments, but that's my aim. If you find the day beneficial, you can practice the day or half-day on a monthly or perhaps quarterly basis.

The type of silence practiced on a day of mindfulness is sometimes called "noble silence," a concept originally from Buddhism. It's noble in the sense of being an admirable practice to engage in. Noble silence is about giving a rest to all your senses, not just your ears. So you turn off the TV, radio, and telephone. You can stop reading and writing and surfing the Internet. All obvious and subtle distractions are put aside. Instead, you open your eyes, ears, and heart to the world around you and within you. In this way, your mind naturally begins to settle, just like the mud settles in a glass of dirty water when you stop shaking it. This is the practice of deep silence and is the spirit of a day of mindfulness. In deep silence, you make space for your body, mind, and heart to heal and nourish themselves.

When I say silence, I mean that you refrain from speaking to anyone. You can be in a place that may not be silent. You can also listen to guided meditations to help structure your practice.

Preparing for a Day of Silent Mindfulness Practice

Choose a day when no one else is at home. If that's not possible, you'll need to let others know not to disturb you as you're doing a "mindfulness experiment" for a day. Rewarding those who don't disturb you with delicious cookies is always well received!

The day before, decide what meals you're going to eat. Ensure you have all the food and drink you need. It's not a problem if the meals require cooking, as preparing and eating food is a wonderful mindfulness practice.

I make sure I don't need to do any work on my day of mindfulness. I certainly keep my laptop closed on that day and my phones off.

Other forms of work that involve the use of your senses can be used in a day of mindfulness. Here are some that offer lots of opportunity to develop mindful awareness:

- Cooking
- Cleaning
- Gardening
- Sweeping
- Ironing

Whether you get a little cooking or cleaning done or not makes no difference. If you think you'll go into doing mode during the activities above, refrain from them.

You'll need some form of timer to indicate the end of each meditation practice. Avoid using your mobile phone for this because you may be tempted to check messages.

Reading anything beyond the odd poem or story based on mindfulness is not recommended. Reading is effectively reentering the world of thoughts, words, and ideas. Instead, give your mind and heart a break from such matters and cultivate a more direct observing perspective of each moment in the day.

You can practice a day of mindfulness on your own or with a friend, group of friends, or family members. The power of practicing mindfulness together in silence can be profound. And you could then explore your experience of the day with each other to share insights.

A Word about Expectations

Consider letting go of all expectations for the day. If you expect the day to be relaxing, calming, and peaceful, you may end up disappointed. And if you expect the day is going to be tough, challenging, and hard work, you may never start. So let go of expectations—just have an open mind and see what happens.

See the day of mindfulness as an experiment on yourself. To see what happens when you take time out just to "be." You did this every day as a baby and young child. You had no agenda, no baggage, no goals. You lived in the present moment. So living a day mindfully isn't alien to you. It's a chance to let go of all the stuff that modern society considers normal and see what happens. Think of it as being like trying out a new hobby or sport and seeing how you find it.

When I first attended a day of mindfulness, I was expecting it to be peaceful, calming, and relaxing. After a few meditations, my back was aching, I was getting irritated by the fidgety person next to me, and I seemed to swing between feeling overly energetic and falling asleep. It was a battle! I was relieved to have made it to the end of the day and thought about never attending another such day. But the week that followed was fascinating. I was calmer and more focused. And things that usually make be feel stressed—my heavy workload and demanding students—were almost nonissues. I wasn't doing anything radically different; my mind was just able to focus easily on one task at a time, and I felt in control. From then on, I let go of all expectations before such a day.

> "I thought eating in silence would be boring. It turned out to feel relaxing and enjoyable. I've never tasted food properly before. It's amazing what misconceptions our brains come up with about a day of silence."

How to Use This Chapter

It's best to read through this whole chapter first and then practice the day of mindfulness at some point this week. If you don't have time to practice the day this week, whenever you can is fine. You could even have a day of mindfulness after the course if you wish.

One way to plan the day would be to use a paper and pen to create a schedule of your day while you read through the recommendations in this chapter. You can use that schedule on the day of mindfulness to guide you, rather than having to read this chapter.

If you're doing the mini-course, you don't need to do a day of mindfulness unless you want to.

> VARIATION: If you're feeling adventurous, why not go with the flow? Just do whatever mindfulness practice or exercise you feel like, and let the day unfold naturally. That can be more fun. If you're the kind of person who loves controlling everything, this would be a great experiment for you—don't plan the day and see what happens.

A Sample Schedule for You

Following is a structure you might use for your day. The timing is approximate—choose times to wake up, sleep, and practice meditation that are realistic for you.

8:00 A.M.: WAKING UP

Ideally, you went to bed early the night before. I personally don't use an alarm, especially on a day of mindfulness, but it's up to you. If you allow yourself to wake up naturally, you'll feel more rested as you'll be waking up at the end of your natural sleep cycle.

Start your day with a mindful pause. A short meditation helps to set the tone for the whole day. Spending a few minutes reflecting on what you're grateful for is also a positive start to your day of mindfulness.

8:15 A.M.: SHOWER

I like to take a shower in the morning, but you can have a bath if you prefer. Not sure how to be mindful in the shower? Simply connect with your senses, any one that you prefer. You could listen to the sound of the water gushing out of the shower or the soft touch of the soap against your warm skin, or the scent of shower gel. Choose any sense and switch between senses as you prefer.

8:30 A.M.: GETTING DRESSED

Getting dressed is something most people do automatically. Today, notice how you choose which clothes to wear. How you wear them in the same way. How you habitually take your time or rush—what do you do? Challenge yourself to notice something different in your dressing routine. Remember to pause before and after getting dressed for a few moments too.

9:00 A.M.: MINDFUL YOGA

Yoga is a great way to start your day of mindfulness. The stretching will help to dispel any morning sleepiness and may make your muscles a bit more relaxed for your meditations in seated postures later.

You can choose to use the mini or full yoga practice in Chapter 13. Use the guided audio if you can't remember all the postures.

9.30 A.M.: MINDFUL EATING

Take your time preparing breakfast. As you go from your yoga to prepare your food, notice the transition. Feel your feet on the floor as you walk and feel the handle on any door that you open.

Prepare your meal with attention in each moment. If you're preparing a fruit salad for yourself, notice the color of the fruit. As you chop an apple, for example, feel the edge of the knife as it cuts through the apple. Hear the sound of the knife cutting through the apple. Take a moment to smell the freshly chopped apple. If you're cooking oatmeal, watch how the consistency changes as you warm the mixture in your saucepan. Listen to the oatmeal as it begins to bubble. Watch the wisps of steam rising up from the pan.

Once your meal is prepared, take some time to set the table. The ritual of setting the table beautifully can enhance your experience of mindfulness. Anything that's different from your habitual way of preparing breakfast will increase your level of mindful awareness.

As you sit down to eat your meal, take a mindful pause. At the end of the pause, take some time to be grateful for the meal in front of you. Remember there are many people who are not as privileged as you and would love such a meal. Take a few moments to look at your breakfast before taking your first bite. Notice how hungry you are. Put your utensil down and enjoy the flavors. Once you've fully chewed and swallowed that first bite, you can go for your second bite and so on. Bring your mind gently back to the meal each time your mind wanders, just like in any other meditation. Notice how your stomach gradually fills up. After you finish your meal, take another few moments to practice a mindful pause.

Eat until you're 80% full: Try *hara hachi bu*

Experiment with eating until you're 80% full. This principle, called *hara hachi bu*, is followed by the Okinawans in Japan. The Okinawans have among the highest number of centenarians (more than 100 years old) in the world, due in part to their lower intake of calories.

As your stomach takes 10–20 minutes to register that it's full, when you think you're about 80% full, you're actually more like 100% full.

Here's how:

1. Begin your meal with a mindful pause, or even just a few mindful breaths.
2. Use a small plate and take the amount of food that you think would leave you about 80% full. Just estimate. I usually take too much food, so for me, it's about taking about 80% of my usual plateful.
3. Eat as mindfully as you can. Connect with the subtle flavors. Count at least 10 chews before swallowing each morsel. Eat with your nondominant hand to help turn off automatic eating. Savor your food and eat with gratitude.
4. Once you've finished the plate, ask yourself: How full am I?
5. If you think you're less than 80% full, go ahead and take a bit more food. But see if you can resist eating until totally full—that point when you feel bloated.

I would call *hara hachi bu* a mindful form of eating as you're tuning in to how full your stomach is rather than eating on autopilot just to finish the plate of food. It also helps you manage a healthy weight. I've been using *hara hachi bu* for the last few months and have lost a few extra pounds—give it a try. I'm not perfect and certainly get a bit carried away in some meals. Just remember to go easy on yourself. If you do automatically overeat, forgiving yourself by saying to yourself, "It's okay. Everyone overeats from time to time," reduces the chance of an emotional binge.

10:15 A.M.: WASHING THE DISHES

I never used to like washing dishes. But with mindfulness, it's far more enjoyable. After a long day working on a computer or in meetings, washing the dishes is a nice, simple activity that can help bring me back into the present moment.

Children love washing dishes. They like feeling the warm water and the bubbles, the magical rainbow of colors as the light catches the soap suds, and the sense of getting a good job done. So bring this sense of seeing things afresh, like a child, when you wash the dishes.

Notice the color of the plate before and after you wash it. Hear the sound of the water from the tap. Really feel the warmth of the water as it softly touches your skin. Experience a few of your breaths from time to time. Wonder at the dexterity of your hands as you lift and wash the dishes without breaking them, which even the most advanced robot can't do at the moment.

10:30 A.M.: MINDFULNESS OF BREATH MEDITATION

In your first meditation practice, start with the simple mindfulness of breath. Set your timer for about 30 minutes.

You can sit either on a chair or on a meditation stool or cushion, whatever feels more comfortable for you. If you want to be reminded how to do mindfulness of breath meditation, see Chapter 5.

11:00 A.M.: MINDFUL WALKING

Walking slowly is great for digestion and reduces sleepiness in your meditation practice. Use Chapter 6 to guide you.

You may like to do mindful walking in your garden. If you're going to walk down the street mindfully, try walking closer to your normal pace and give full attention in each moment as best you can. If you're very close to a park or other natural surroundings, try walking there to enhance your experience.

11:30 A.M.: EXPANDING AWARENESS MEDITATION

Once you return from your walk, you can go straight into this meditation. Rather than having lots of guidance, practice with just bells (audio tracks 21–24) to indicate that you need to move from one stage (e.g., mindfulness of breath) to another (e.g., mindfulness of body).

As the day progresses, using less audio guidance and having more silence is an effective way to help deepen your meditation. Although guidance is helpful for pacing and reminding you to bring your attention back, for some people it acts like a distraction from being fully attentive to their unfolding present-moment experience.

NOON: MOUNTAIN OR LAKE MEDITATION

These are guided-imagery-type meditations, which are not typical in mindfulness practice. However, I've come to discover that some people really enjoy this type of meditation, and it helps to make mindfulness more accessible to them.

The purpose of these meditations is to help you understand the practice of mindfulness at a deeper level. They act as metaphors, pointing you to ways of accessing greater degrees of stability, groundedness, inner strength, and acceptance and to reflect on your inner sense of wholeness despite the seeming transience of the world.

Choose whichever one appeals to you or do them both if you have time.

Tales of Wisdom: The Moon Can't Be Stolen

Once a thief clambered through the window and into a meditation master's home. He searched around frantically but couldn't find anything of value to steal. Frustrated, as he was about to leave, the meditation master heard a noise and went downstairs. He saw the thief and said, "Are you leaving empty-handed?" The thief froze, bemused by the comment. Finally he replied, "Yes . . . why?" "Let me give you some clothes!" remarked the teacher. He handed over a small pile of clothes. The thief thought the guy was crazy! He took the clothes and ran out. The teacher stepped out of his home, walked to a nearby lake, and smiled as he watched the pale moon just above the horizon. "If only I could give him the moon," he thought.

PRACTICE: Mountain Meditation

Audio track 18: About 20 minutes.

Here's the guidance for the mountain meditation:

1. Sit in a posture that is upright, balanced, and still, without straining your back. Allow your eyes to close gently or softly cast your eyes downward.
2. Take three deep, full in- and out-breaths, feeling each breath as you do so. Then let your breath find its own natural rhythm.
3. Spend a few minutes feeling your breathing. Notice you're watching the body breathing itself. You don't actually have to do anything.
4. When you're ready, bring to mind the image of a beautiful, majestic mountain. It may be one that you've seen before or one that you made up in your imagination, or perhaps a combination of the two.
5. Take your time to imagine this picture. Allow the image of the mountain to come slowly into focus. Don't worry if you don't think you're a visual person. Just do the best you can, which is absolutely fine.
6. Stay aware of the image of the mountain. What color is it? Does it have snow on its peak? Notice the shape of the mountain with its peak up high in the sky, perhaps above the clouds. Notice how the base of your mountain is firmly fixed on the earth's surface. Are there any trees growing on the slopes? What sort of natural vegetation do you notice?
7. As you see this mountain as best you can, be aware of its stability. How grounded the mountain is. Really feel the presence of the mountain—as if it's right here in front of you.
8. Now allow yourself to merge into the mountain. So, in a sense, you are the mountain. Your head is the lofty peak of the mountain. The sides of your body are the slopes of this beautiful mountain. And the seat you're sitting on is where the mountain becomes one with the rest of the earth. You share the immense size, stillness, and majesty of the mountain. And you, as the mountain, view the panoramic vista around you.
9. Your buttocks and legs represent the mountain rooted to the earth. Feel a gentle uplift in your posture, starting deep within your pelvis and spine, upright just like that mountain.

10. You sit as if you are a breathing mountain. Still, serene, centered, and majestic. Your presence has qualities beyond thought and words.

11. As you sit here as the mountain, you notice the sun moving across the sky, continuing changing areas of color, light, and shade. And eventually day turns to night. Overhead is a roof made of stars and wispy clouds and the bright, pale moon, casting its silver light in its own delicate way. And night eventually gives way to dawn, and a new day with new possibilities and subtly different experiences.

12. Different days bring different weather. Some days cloudy, other days clear. Sometimes it rains and you see the most beautiful rainbow. Other days, bright sunlight. And through all this change that surrounds you, you remain the same. Dignified, solid, and fully centered in the present.

13. As the days pass, the seasons change. In summer the sun may melt most of the snow. Any trees on the slope filling up with leaves and nature are a flurry of activity. In fall, the temperatures cool and the leaves may turn into a fiery orange. With winter may come snow, cool winds, and more clouds. This is a time for rest and hibernation for much of nature. And as winter gradually blends into spring, the activity of nature begins again.

14. All this change makes no difference to you in your essence as the mountain. You're familiar with change and accept this to be the way things are. You also know your inner being to be still, calm, solid, beyond thought, and one with the earth itself. You just sit, even when buffeted by the most violent of storms, with its wind and rain.

15. Just as the mountain experiences changes in each day and season, so you have different experiences with each day and season. And sometimes you are faced with violent storms in your body and mind. Tuning in to the essence of the mountain can remind you that there is a place within you that remains centered and still despite the seemingly huge changes that surround you.

16. The way through life's changes and challenges is opening up with awareness. There is no experience that awareness cannot hold. In your willingness and courage to feel the cold wind and violent storms, you simultaneously open awareness to the possibility that the storm will pass—that moment by moment, change will occur and there will be another spring after winter.

17. Your internal weather may include draining thoughts, difficult emotions, and painful sensations. But the mountain doesn't take the weather personally. The mountain doesn't hold any grudge. The weather is simply weathering. Perhaps your internal weather is impersonal too, and

part and parcel of the nature of things. A resistance to those experiences is just adding to the suffering, which takes time to see.

18. The weather of your life is not to be ignored. Instead, you can discover the value of honoring and respecting the weather and come to see that the awareness that holds it is also in some mysterious way peaceful and free of it.

19. If you found some value in reflecting on the qualities of a mountain, to bring you to an inner stillness, vitality, and stability, you can bring this image to mind in your meditations and daily life.

20. Continue to practice sitting, being with your breathing and bodily sensations, until it is time for you to stop.

PRACTICE: Lake Meditation

Audio track 19: About 20 minutes.

Here's the guidance for the lake meditation:

1. Begin by finding a place to lie down. You can use a mat on the floor or lie on a bed. Allow your eyes to close. Take a few deep, slow breaths and then just feel your breath as it finds its own natural rhythm.

2. When you're ready, bring to mind, and to heart, the image of a beautiful lake. It may be a lake you've seen long ago, etched in your memory. Or it may be a lake that you just make up in your imagination, perhaps based on a postcard or painting that you've seen. As best you can, notice the color of the lake—is it crystal clear or a little muddy? What's the size and shape of the lake? Does the still surface of the lake reflect the backdrop, which may be mountains or trees or clouds that are gliding elegantly through the clear blue sky? If it's windy, notice how it whips up the surface of the water, creating diamonds of light as they catch the sunlight. And yet deep underneath, the water is still and calm, supporting the movement above. And as day turns to the stillness of night, and the wind calms, you may be able to see a canopy of dazzling stars and the majesty of the moon glowing on the earth. As the seasons change, which they inevitably and effortlessly do, the lake may freeze over, surrounded by a blanket of snow like icing, heavily dusted on a cake.

3. As you lie here, breathing, and when you're ready to do so, allow your

mind and heart and being to merge with the lake. So you are, in some way, this magnificent lake. As a living, breathing lake you reflect the beauty of your natural surroundings and the ever-changing sky above.

4. As you continue to breathe, notice how the earth forms a solid basin, holding the lake in stillness. The lake seems to just accept the days, nights, seasons, and years that go by. And in that lack of resistance, in that letting go, lies the beauty of the lake. As you lie here, what thoughts and feelings and sensations are you willing to accept and let go as the reality of this moment? Can you reflect them as they are, just as the lake does?

5. Notice how the lake is the same in some ways, and in some ways ever changing. In the same way, notice how each present moment is different and yet the awareness that is underlying all your experiences creates a sense of safe familiarity.

6. As the wind rises and falls, the surface of the lake is disturbed. And as storms make their bold appearance, the still lake may seem a distant memory. But deep underneath the lake, there's another story. Another viewpoint. There's more to the lake than just the surface. Near the base of the lake are calm, peaceful waters. As your mind tosses and turns and your emotions create giant ripples in your life, can you remember this lake? Can you see beyond the surface? Your base, your being, the heart of awareness itself, remains unchanged, solid, still, and supportive.

7. You may like to bring this metaphor of the lake to mind whenever you face storms in your life, with the intensity of thoughts and emotions that they bring. You can also use the lake metaphor in your meditations, to enrich and deepen your practice in some way.

8. As you lie here, feeling your breathing and opening up to feeling your body as a whole, rest as the lake does. Open your mind and heart to the richness of your surroundings, accepting each moment as it is. Reflecting sun and clouds, trees and mountains, birds and butterflies. Mirroring mist and fog and cloud and dust. And as your waters lap against the shores in the coolness of night, tune in to that quiet stillness, that wonder and mystery of those millions of stars, all reflected, without effort and with reverence, in this lake that is within you.

9. Continue to practice tuning in to this lake, moment by moment, until you are ready to bring this meditation to a close. And finish by remembering to honor your efforts to practice today, to cultivate awareness and compassion for yourself and thereby create positive ripples in all those you meet.

12:30 P.M.: YOGA

You can do either yoga sequence in Chapter 13. If you find guidance helpful for pacing, support, or to remind you how to do the postures, use the full yoga audio. If you remember how to do the postures, you are welcome to practice them without the audio, using whatever postures and stretches your body needs now.

"This will sound a bit crazy, but I had a feeling of being one with everything in one of the meditations. It felt so restful—just a minute in that state felt like a full night of deep sleep. The ultimate feeling of letting go. That was a nice side effect of the day of mindfulness!"

Tune in to the more subtle sensations and messages from your body as you practice yoga. Remember, feeling your breathing is a key part of mindful yoga. And be compassionate with your own body, being careful not to push past your physical limits.

1:00 P.M.: LUNCH

Prepare your lunch in the same mindful way as was described for breakfast. Take your time to prepare, eat, and wash up afterwards, pausing after each activity to gather your attention and center yourself in the here and now.

2:00 P.M.: MINDFUL WALKING OR A NAP

This afternoon, experiment with the following mindful walking exercise if you can.

PRACTICE: Mindful Slow and Fast Walking

1. Begin your mindful walking at your normal pace. Notice the sensations of your feet on the floor or the touch of air against your skin. Alternatively, you could tune in to the sensation of your breath as you walk.

2. Now become aware of your thoughts and feelings as you walk. Notice them and, as best you can, watch them from a distance rather than getting caught up in them.

3. Next, increase your walking pace and clench your fists and jaw. Sense what the extra tension feels like. Notice what thoughts and feelings arise for you this time.

4. Release the tension in your body, but continue to walk at a faster pace. Hold your head upright and chest open. Note how this feels. What thoughts arise this time?

5. Gradually go back to your normal pace of walking. Find that natural rhythm and tune in to your bodily sensations as you walk.

6. Now stop. Observe your bodily sensations. Notice your heartbeat, the temperature of your body, and the rate of your breathing. Move the spotlight of your awareness into your inner world of thoughts and emotions—place your thoughts on imaginary clouds if that helps.

7. Begin walking more slowly, staying mindful of each step. Slowly walk back to where you started.

8. Finish in the mountain posture (see Chapter 13), tuning in to your inner experiences and reflecting on what you observed in this exercise, without judgment.

The change of pace and tension help to energize you after lunch and allow you to see the effect of the body on the mind and emotions, as well as vice versa.

If you feel tired after lunch, you could also take a nap for 20–30 minutes. It'll help reset your circadian cycle, which is designed for a short snooze in the early afternoon, and you'll feel fresher rather than fighting fatigue later on. If you sleep too much, you may feel groggy, so watch out for that.

2:45 P.M.: EXPANDING AWARENESS MEDITATION

Practice the expanding awareness meditation in Chapter 8, either by yourself or using the audio if you need it. As you've been practicing mindfulness for a few hours now, it's particularly beneficial to practice with extended periods of silence. The silence helps you tune in to your own, subtle experiences in each moment.

Audio track 22—silence with bells every 5 minutes.

To do this, use the audio, which is silence with just bells.

3:15 P.M.: CULTIVATING COMPASSION: LOVING-KINDNESS MEDITATION

Compassion cultivates the desire to relieve the suffering in others. It is about knowing that both you and others go through difficulties in life and have the desire to end that suffering.

This meditation is a powerful exercise to do toward the end of your day of mindfulness. This is because when your mind is calmer, you are better able to access and cultivate feelings of friendliness toward yourself and others.

One way of cultivating compassion is through the "loving-kindness meditation," which is described below. Loving-kindness meditation can help you move from isolation to connection, from judgment to caring, and from dislike to understanding. You don't need to force any emotion to arise. That is a common misunderstanding. Simply give your attention and authentic well-wishing in each phrase you say to yourself and see what arises. Think of yourself like an open field, in which you're planting seeds of compassion. As with all meditations, don't worry if your mind keeps wandering or wanders off for long periods of time. Guide that attention back as softly and smoothly as you can, when you can.

You can use the audio to guide you through it and can make use of it after you finish the course.

PRACTICE: Loving-Kindness Meditation

Audio track 20: 30 minutes.

1. For this meditation, ensure you're feeling particularly comfortable and warm. The physical feeling of safety and warmth will help to cultivate the emotional quality of compassion. You can be seated comfortably or lie down if you wish.

2. Take a few deep, slow, mindful breaths. Then let your body find its own natural flow of breath. Feel your breathing in the area near your heart. Notice whether your chest is rising and falling. Be aware of the warmth of your body. Try placing your hand, representing self-kindness and care, softly on your heart area and notice what effect that has. Feel the warmth of your hand on your heart. If you prefer to place your hand on your belly or your lap, that's fine too.

3. When you're ready, bring to mind someone, or even a pet, that makes you smile. Someone with whom you have an easy and positive relationship. Perhaps not your partner, as such relationships tend to be complex and it's easy to get lost in thoughts. Maybe an aunt or uncle, perhaps your young son or daughter, a spiritual figure, or another person you hold in great respect, whether the person is alive or not. Wish this person well with words like:

Research Corner: Why Practice Compassion?

Scientists have found when you feel compassion, your heart rate slows down, you release a hormone called oxytocin that promotes bonding, and the part of your brain involved in care and pleasure is activated. You are then motivated to care for and help others. Compassion also increases resilience to stress and boosts the immune system to accelerate healing.

You can train yourself to be more and more compassionate with practice—it's not a fixed trait, but more like a muscle. Researchers at Emory University have found people who did a compassion training course had greater levels of compassion and lower levels of stress hormones in their blood and saliva.

Self-compassion in particular trumps self-esteem. Research by Kristin Neff found that people with high self-esteem could end up in traps like narcissism, self-righteous anger, prejudice, and self-absorption. Consider those who have high self-esteem and see themselves as high achievers. This self-image can cause them to believe they are above others, and their arrogance comes at a cost: when things go wrong in life, their self-esteem naturally drops as their self-image as superior crumbles. This is a stressful way to live.

Self-compassion, in contrast, is about being kind to yourself and seeing your imperfection as human. With this tendency, you'll refrain from criticizing yourself and not be vulnerable to seeing yourself as worth less when things go wrong. You'll have greater resilience against future life challenges and therefore lower levels of stress.

I experienced self-esteem issues myself. For example, when I was a high school student, I was top in the class. My sense of self-esteem was high, built on my academic achievements. But in university, I never achieved the highest grade in the class. The more I tried, the more frustrated I got. I felt low and wanted to give up. By good fortune, I discovered mindfulness halfway through my studies. I learned the value of self-compassion and finished my studies successfully without pushing myself too hard.

Other fascinating recent studies have found compassion to heal, but empathy to hurt. Empathy is a way to feel other people's suffering but can lead to emotional burnout. For example, health professionals or caregivers can become distressed themselves and suffer greatly. Empathy activates areas in the brain associated with unpleasant feelings like sadness and pain. Compassion is very different. Compassion activates the more warm and caring parts of the brain, like a loving mother toward her crying baby.

World-renowned Buddhist monk Matthieu Ricard has been collaborating with several scientists, including Tania Singer, neuroscientist and Director of the Department of Social Neuroscience at the Max Planck Institute. Their research, published in 2014 in the journal *Social Cognitive and Affective Neuroscience*, suggests that those in the helping professions should do compassion training to help protect them from empathy burnout. Watch this space!

"May you be happy, may you be healthy,
and may you be free from suffering."

Allow the words to sound in your heart area rather than your head, if you can. Tune in to both the words and the meaning behind the words. And if some other words resonate with you, use them. Use words that represent kindness and compassion for you. Continue repeating these words for a few minutes. Remember, you don't need to force any feelings at all—just wish wellness and make space for any feelings to arise.

4. Now, in the same spirit, bring yourself to mind. Wish yourself well. You are just as worthy as any other being on the planet. You deserve an equal amount of kindness and care.

"May I be happy. May I be healthy. May I be filled
with compassion and kindness towards myself.
May I be free from suffering."

This is the most difficult stage for some people. You may feel guilty for sending kindness to yourself, or think you're overindulging yourself. If this is the case, this stage of the loving-kindness meditation is going to be a useful exercise for you to help relieve stress. Stress can often be heightened by being too hard on yourself, and this meditation is a great antidote. If you felt a resistance to self-kindness, that's okay. Given time, this will be a particularly nourishing and healing meditation for you. Try to be patient as best you can. Persevere gently and notice what happens with interest.

5. Next, bring to mind a neutral person—someone you neither like nor dislike, someone you hardly know. For example, someone at the toll booth, the supermarket checkout, or the mail carrier. Remember that they, like you, have a life outside their work role. Consider their friends and family, their hopes and fears, desires and dreams. Wish them well. Use your own words or use these:

"May you be happy and healthy. May you be filled
with love and peace. May you be free from all pain
and suffering."

6. Next up is someone you don't like—a difficult person. This person may be dead or alive. As a beginner, choose someone who's quite

difficult, but not the most difficult person you know. It may be some-one who has caused you problems and suffering in the past. Consider him or her as a whole person, beyond just the hurt the person caused you. As a human being, this person also experiences pain, anxiety, stress, and a host of difficulties. See if you can forgive his actions, which he may have done unknowingly. And if the pain inflicted on you was deliberate, perhaps there was a reason—the person's emotional state, his own vulnerability and pain, his needs being unfulfilled. If you can, ask the person to forgive you for any hurt you caused him too. You're not assuming what he did was right, just letting go of the pain caused by his actions. This warms your heart instead of hardening it.

> "May you be well and happy and healthy. May you be
> free of stress, anxiety, pain. May your heart be filled
> with self-kindness and compassion."

7. Bring to mind all four of you: yourself, your friend, your neutral per-son, and your difficult person. As you imagine all of you together, see if you can offer a sense of well-wishing and compassion to all, equally.
8. You can finish this meditation by offering loving-kindness to all beings on the planet—being mindful of the difficulties and suffering that all beings face and wishing them to be free of that suffering.
9. Now come back to yourself. Center your attention on your breath-ing, feeling its natural pace and depth. Bring a sense of warmth, affection, and gratitude to your breath.
10. Before you end the meditation, appreciate your efforts to cultivate one of life's most nourishing qualities—compassion.

VARIATION: You can practice this loving-kindness meditation at any time after you finish this course. And you don't need to do all the stages if you don't have time. You can do just one or two or whichever stage you feel you need to.

4:00 P.M.: MINDFUL DAILY ACTIVITY

Start by having a drink and/or snack if you need it. During this time period, spend time gardening, cleaning, sweeping outside, or going for a walk. You may like to take the time to lie in bed and sleep if you're feeling very tired. Check in with your body and see what your body needs.

6:00 P.M.: PREPARING AND EATING DINNER MINDFULLY

Follow the same principles as for breakfast and lunch.

7:30 P.M.: BATHING OR MINDFUL ACTIVITIES

Listening to music can be a nice way to bring the day of mindfulness to a close. Play a piece of music and lie down and just allow the sounds to enter your ears and go deeply into your being. I'd recommend classical or other calming forms of music. Alternatively, you may enjoy some simple painting, a gentle evening walk, tending to your plants, or some yoga.

You may also like to take a nice relaxing bath. This can be combined with lighting a few candles. Use the opportunity to connect with your senses rather than just allow your mind to drift. Smell the scent of the bath salts, observe the flickering candles, notice the sensations in your body as your muscles slowly begin to relax in the warm water. Listening to the sound of the water as it fills up the bath is also another very pleasant and mindful exercise.

8:30 P.M.: FINAL MEDITATION OF THE DAY

Finish the day with a meditation of your choice—sitting meditation or body scan.

9:30 P.M.: BEDTIME ROUTINE AND SLEEP

Get ready for bed, paying attention to your habitual routine. Then lie down, gently close your eyes, and feel your whole body as you lie in bed. Take a few moments to scan through your body from head to toe. Observe whether your body feels different from how it normally feels at the end of the day. Feel your breathing as it finds its natural rhythm. Continue this gentle mindful awareness until you eventually drift off into sleep.

Reflection

The day after your day of mindfulness, write down what you noticed. What was challenging? What aspects did you enjoy? If you were to have such a day again, what changes would you make to enhance your experience?

Drink from That Well

I begin today with anticipation,
To savor a different kind of way,
Yet find myself in isolation,
Emotions grip me in disarray

But there is inside me a deeper cry,
For peace and silence and calm and joy.
And though the clock says hours to go,
I smile, and remember, this breath is all!

Beneath the surface, attention-seeking waves,
That we call thoughts, moods, sensations, tough days.
I long to feel, to be with, to love,
To reclaim sweet clarity of a pure white dove.

Now I'm ready to start again.
To be me, myself, to sit, to rest.
Not rest in sleep, in slumber, or dwell.
But rest in awareness,
And drink from that well.

—SHAMASH ALIDINA

Reflection:
Discoveries from Week 6 Home Experiments

Take a few moments to reflect on your daily mindful communication—your daily mindful booster this week. How did that go? Did you actually manage to remember to communicate mindfully, once a day? Many people forget, as automatic pilot mode is the default in the human brain. If you forgot, notice that—no need to berate yourself. Instead, see this as a chance to learn just how automatic we humans can be! If you did manage to remember, how was the experience? Did you notice yourself rushing through the conversation, or feeling impatient? Did you find yourself tempted to multitask as you spoke?

Recall the story of the three questions (Chapter 6)—the most important person is the person who's in front of you. It doesn't matter whether it's a princess or a pauper; consider whoever is in front of you as the most important person in the world who is worthy of your full attention. Listening to this person fully is one of the greatest meditations.

Jot down any reflections on mindful communication in your journal or digital device.

Day of Mindfulness FAQs

Q: I felt emotional and found myself crying. Is that normal?

A: Feeling emotional and crying is absolutely normal during a day of mindfulness. You may never have taken so much extended time in quiet rather than being distracted. This spaciousness can give permission for your body to release any pent-up or suppressed emotions. It's a good thing and nothing that you need to worry about. I've heard many stories of people being healed of physical illnesses after an emotional release in a meditation retreat. For example, one client overcame her chronic headaches after a retreat. Another client had shoulder pain for a couple of years, but it went away after a retreat.

Q: I found the day emotionally and physically draining. I actually feel more tired now. What did I do wrong?

A: You didn't do anything wrong. As explained earlier, a day of mindfulness can create an emotional state for people. Emotions are there to be felt rather than pushed away or ignored. The day of mindfulness gives you a safe opportunity to practice being with emotions within yourself. If you feel that the emotions are overwhelming for you, perhaps you need to see a health professional to see other ways of getting help with managing your emotions. The day of mindfulness can be draining physically as well. A range of practices like expanding awareness meditation with yoga and walking can help reduce the physical toll on your body. However, part of the physical drain can be linked to the emotions that are released. Be gentle with yourself as best you can and see if you can avoid too much intense activity on the day following the day of mindfulness. The positive effects from a day of mindfulness may not be observed consciously and may be taking place unconsciously within your mind and heart. These processes take time rather than being an immediate fix. One of my clients didn't seem to gain any benefit—just felt waves of anger come and go. He almost left during the day out of frustration. But in the days that followed, he found himself better able to spot moments of self-criticism when at work; he was more mindful of his thought patterns. He was then able to say kinder words to himself rather than berate himself so much. This reduced his stress significantly.

Q: How often should I have a day of mindfulness?

A: As often as you wish. Having two or three days of mindfulness in a year is a good start. But if you have time to practice more, that's absolutely fine! Evidence seems to suggest the more you practice mindfulness the more benefits you accrue. You could have the odd morning or afternoon of mindfulness whenever you have time, too.

Q: I've heard of people going for a weekend of mindfulness or even a one-week retreat. Do you recommend that?

A: Yes, I do recommend longer periods of mindfulness practice if you're willing to do it. However, begin with a few one-day mindfulness sessions and then build up to the weekend before going on to do a full week of silent mindfulness. That way you are less likely to put yourself off from doing the extended mindfulness retreats in the future.

Q: I couldn't do a whole day of mindfulness, in silence! Why should I force myself to do that?!

A: There's no need to force yourself to do anything. If you're happy just doing the little mindfulness exercises and meditations, that's fine. If you ever feel you'd like to discover more about your own mind and heart, then experiment with a couple of hours of mindfulness—maybe the body scan, expanding awareness meditation, and some mindful walking. And build up to a day of mindfulness if you feel inclined to do so. You're allowed to take your time and come to a day of mindfulness, when you're ready and choose to do so.

ELEVEN

Week 7

Taking Care of Yourself

If someone comes along and shoots an arrow into your heart, it's fruitless to stand there and yell at the person. It would be much better to turn your attention to the fact that there's an arrow in your heart.

—PEMA CHÖDRÖN

INTENTIONS

+ *To adjust your lifestyle to reduce stress.*
+ *To identify your nourishing and depleting activities.*
+ *To develop a mindful stress management action plan.*
+ *To discover what a "mindful action step" is.*

NOT LONG AGO a young woman named Valentina applied for one of my online training programs and told me on the phone a lot about her background. She said that after experiencing a string of traumatic events she was so racked with panic and agony that she turned to an array of drugs to try to numb her emotions. Eventually she reached the proverbial rock bottom, with no friends or family willing to continue a relationship with her.

Miraculously, one day she discovered an uncashed check made out to her for a sizable sum, and this presented her with a choice. Describing her decision as flowing from a rare moment of clarity, she invested in rehab instead of funding her addictions. At the rehab center she happened upon a stone bench beside a stream and felt inexplicably drawn to it. Without knowing that what she was doing was actually a form of meditation, she sat cross-legged on the bench and listened to the trickling water with her eyes closed, in the midst of a peaceful silence that instantly felt healing.

For Valentina, this was the first step on the road to mindfulness, self-compassion, and new self-awareness honed through meditation practice and daily journaling. As she described her transformation from a hard-drinking, drugging hedonist to a sober vegan yogi, she laughed boisterously and marveled at the fact that people—including those who had once found her impossible to be around—now often point out how cheerful and open she is. Quietly then, Valentina said she thought her friendly personality combined with her difficult history would make her a dedicated, empathetic mindfulness teacher.

I did, of course, accept Valentina into the course.

In one transformative moment, Valentina chose life rather than the path to self-destruction, and that was an act of self-care. From that important fork in the road, I'm sure there were many moments of choice where she could have gone back to her old lifestyle. But she got through, using mindfulness. That initial choice has led her to eat healthy food, exercise, practice meditation and yoga, and spend time with good company. This kind of nourishing lifestyle has borne such powerful fruit that she has the energy, enthusiasm, and love to share her discoveries with others. Her self-care and self-compassion are spilling over into care and compassion for others in her original predicament. Without caring for herself, this would be impossible.

Looking After Yourself

There are probably many demands on your time and energy, and looking after yourself can easily slip down the to-do list. Perhaps you're a busy mom, a pressured business executive, or recently bereaved. When faced with lots of demands, it's easy to forget to take care of yourself. When you do look after yourself, your feelings of distress begin to turn into positive eustress (see Chapter 7), and you're better able to meet life's challenges with a smile.

Take a moment to think about how caring owners treat their dog. They wash and groom him, give him sufficient and healthy food, ensure their dog is at the right weight, and exercise the dog every day. They make sure they give their beloved animal time and attention and play games with the dog when out and about. At night they make sure their dog is warm enough and has a place to sleep. So dogs are given food, exercise, fun, love, and rest. And in return the dog gives unconditional love to the owner. We humans also need at least the same sort of love and care to meet life's challenges with enthusiasm and hope.

Before you start thinking how little you take care of yourself, take a few moments to reflect on how much your body already looks after you. All day and night, your body breathes for you. Your heart beats over 100,000 times in a day to pump blood containing oxygen, nutrients, and immune cells around your body. Your digestive system processes 1,100 pounds of food a year. Your body urges you to eat, sleep, and move around to keep you alive and well. So in all these many ways, your body is taking care of you.

But you have a role to play too. Taking care of yourself involves eating a balanced diet, sleeping sufficiently, and exercising your body. And just as important, you need to make time for socializing, having fun, and doing things you enjoy. Exactly what you need to do to look after yourself is unique to you, and only you can know what the right choices are. By being more aware of your body and mind, you can learn to take better care of yourself.

For example, one client of mine started getting painful spots on his legs. He tried to ignore them and carried on with his high-pressure job. Eventually they became so painful he couldn't walk, and he had to get antibiotics from his doctor and take time off work. Now he's more mindful of his body, and when the spots appear, he needs to make a conscious effort to practice mindfulness and take a little time off. He hasn't suffered from a severe recurrence of the spots ever since.

For you the warning signs may be a headache, a bout with the flu, painful shoulders, or just dwelling on everything that's going wrong in your life. Use these signs to remind you to be kind to yourself rather than pushing harder or reprimanding yourself for not being perfect.

This week you'll have a chance to look at your typical daily activities. You can then identify what, if anything, needs to be adjusted so that you're nourishing your body and mind, not just depleting yourself. You'll also look at a set of five areas to focus on, to help boost your well-being and build resilience against stressors.

The Challenge of Taking Care of Yourself

If looking after ourselves were easy, we would all be doing it well. But in reality, there are challenges that prevent you from taking full care of yourself. Some of them are external factors, and others may just be attitudes in your own mind. Let's look at a few typical challenges and tips to overcome them.

Lack of willpower is rated as the number-one reason we don't take effective care of ourselves, according to the American Psychological Association.

If you know you need to go to bed on time or go for a run, but somehow end up wasting time, you may need some help to boost your self-control. Here are some tips for increasing your willpower:

- **Mindfulness meditation increases willpower.** Even a few minutes a day can start building up gray matter in areas of the brain that control decision making.
- **Exercise.** People who exercise are more likely to quit smoking, reduce alcohol consumption, eat more healthily, and even be more careful with their spending habits.
- **Sleep.** The closer you can get to about 7½ hours of sleep a night, the stronger your willpower will be.
- **Build good habits.** When you're under stress, you go back to your habits, good or bad. So by having good habits, you will be better able to handle or even enjoy the stress.
- **Being nice to yourself really works.** When you lapse, being self-critical reduces your willpower. One of the most well-tested areas in willpower research is that self-compassion is the most effective way to achieve good new habits. Remember that you're only human and can't be perfect.

Lack of time is a common reason people give for not taking care of themselves through measures like exercise or cooking a proper meal. If this is the case for you, I'd recommend you spend a week tracking how you spend your time, hour by hour. When I did this, just the act of setting an alarm every hour and writing down how I was spending my time made me much more efficient. I then managed to get to sleep on time rather than surfing online and exercised rather than working unproductively. Many time management gurus recommend time tracking as the first step toward using time effectively.

If you feel overwhelmed with responsibilities, you may feel too pressured to be able to look after yourself well. But even a 5-minute brisk walk a day can start to create small positive changes in your brain and body to help you cope with the busyness of life.

Finally, you may think of taking care of yourself as being selfish. Recall the safety advice on flights: Always put on your own oxygen mask before doing the same for anyone else. By taking good care of yourself, you'll feel better, have more energy, and be able to help others.

> "Through mindfulness I realized I was constantly running around looking after my kids and husband and parents. I never had time for myself. Never. I immediately decided things have got to change. That's been a huge relief."

I have struggled with this idea myself. When I first became a schoolteacher, I was young, full of energy, and wanted to change the world. I gave all my energy to caring for my students rather than myself. I worked harder and harder until I started to get ill. Not spending my free time working on lesson plans, marking books, or doing extra training seemed selfish. But I started to notice a pattern. The harder I worked, the less energy I had for the kids and the less effective I was as a teacher. On the days I rested well, I had far more patience and the lessons went well. Taking care of myself, even if I felt guilty at first, was better for both my students and me. Nowadays, I love taking care of myself!

When to Take Care of Yourself

Seeing to your own needs is not something you do only when feeling worn out, stressed, or tired. If you do it all the time, as a matter of course, you'll be resilient when the next stressor comes around the corner. However, it's especially important to look after your needs when under excessive stress.

Take plants as an example. In winter, when it's cooler, my plants don't need much watering. Once a week is fine. But in the summer, in the relentless heat, daily watering is necessary. Otherwise the plants will wilt and weaken. When the heat is on, more nourishment is required.

In the same way, when the heat of stress is high, take extra care of yourself. After a stressful day, take a few moments or a few minutes to practice your favorite mindfulness meditation. Try to see the practice as a little treat after a tough day. This may help you go to bed a little earlier, eat a bit healthier, or maybe give you motivation to take time to exercise. Even a 5-minute phone call to your best friend can make a world of difference. A little bit of mindfulness following a challenging day will be an investment that pays back handsomely.

A Look at Your Current Lifestyle

Before you start thinking about how great or poor you are at taking care of yourself, let's start by taking a closer look at your current lifestyle. The activities you do habitually will give you a good idea about what's going well and which areas need tweaking. Until you stop and write this down, you may not realize how you currently use your time.

You'll then rate each activity as either energizing (nourishing) or draining (depleting). This will help you see what proportion of your day is uplifting and what proportion isn't. You can then either look at creative ways of readjusting your schedule or readjusting your attitude and perception so the draining activities aren't quite so draining.

Here's a sample list:

7:00 A.M.—Wake up
7:15 A.M.—Shower and get dressed
7:45 A.M.—Get the kids ready for school
8:30 A.M.—(Rush) to school
9:00 A.M.—Drive to work
9:30 A.M.—Arrive at work
9:45 A.M.—Work on new marketing plan
            And so on . . .

EXERCISE: My Nourishing and Depleting Activities

1. **Create your own daily list** of activities you do in a typical day.
2. **Add a +** for activities that are nourishing, uplifting, or energizing for you. These are the activities that make you feel good.
3. **Add a –** to activities that are depleting or make you feel drained or tired. These are the activities that make you feel worse.
4. **Which positive activities can you do more often?** Go through the list and see which ones you could do more of. For example, going for a walk, reading a story to the kids, waking up a few minutes earlier to have time for a nice cup of coffee.
5. **Which negative activities can you reduce?** For example, cut checking social media sites to only once a day, doing fewer chores by delegating, such as training the children to wash the dishes after dinner, or making some activities less stressful by, for instance, listening to your favorite music on your morning commute.

VARIATION: Compare your thoughts with reality. Record how you felt as soon as you can after doing the activity and how strongly you felt on a scale of 1–10 (1 being very mild and 10 being very intense)—for example, happy 7/10 or annoyed 8/10. See if the activity really was nourishing or depleting for you. For example, people think they enjoy watching television for hours, but when they actually do this, they rate it as just about as interesting as sitting in the bathroom!

GOING DEEPER: If you enjoy this process and want more detail, try recording your daily activities for a full week, including the weekend, to get a clearer picture of what you do. And jot down your mood every hour or so to see if you can spot any patterns.

TIPS Some activities may seem energizing at the time, but later on you find they have depleted your energy. For example, drinking several glasses of wine may seem to make you feel good at the time, but later on in the evening, you may regret it. In that case, you may choose to label it as depleting.

Other activities may feel draining but actually energize you. For example, exercise may feel like it's depleting your energy at the time you do it, but afterward, or perhaps the next day, you may feel more energized.

I recommend you record your feelings as soon as you can after the experience, but look out for these patterns in your journal, described in the drinking and exercise example above.

Reflection

Did you make any new discoveries through this exercise? What changes in your schedule, or perhaps your attitude, can you make? Small changes like that can have a surprisingly big impact.

For example, one of my clients who used to find it depleting to listen to her mother on the phone practiced mindful breathing as she listened. The phone calls became meditation time rather than criticism and fight time, and she felt less overwhelmed by the stress as a result.

Tales of Wisdom: How to Walk on Water

Three monks were sitting by the side of a lake in meditation. Suddenly, the first monk got up and said, "I forgot to put my underwear out to dry!" and miraculously walked on the water, across the lake, and into his hut, before promptly returning.

Before long, the second monk jumped up and said, "I forgot to flush the toilet" and immediately got up and strolled on top of water, into his hut, and came back again, in the same amazing way.

The third monk thought, "These monks think they have some sort of superior meditation technique and are just showing off. I can do that easily. I'm a far better meditator then they'll ever be." The monk stood up, attempted to confidently walk on water, and immediately fell into the lake. He got out, psyched himself up, and tried again. The same thing happened. Before long, he was completely soaked.

The other two monks calmly watched the scene, and then one monk said to the other, "Shall we tell him where the stones are?"

What's the moral of the story for you?

When Stress Overwhelms

The following practice is a three-step exercise you can try using when you feel overwhelmed by stress.

PRACTICE: The Mindful ABC

The exercise is made up of steps A, B, and C to make it easier to remember. A stands for awareness, B stands for breath and beliefs, and C stands for choosing a mindful action, as explained on pages 245–246 and illustrated in the diagram below.

Step A: Awareness
•Notice your stress signs
•Identify your stressors

Step B: Breath and Beliefs
•Feel your breath and body
•Reframe beliefs about the stress or stressor

Step C: Choice
•Accept situation
or
•Change situation

Step A: Awareness

Become aware of your stress signs. These are the thoughts, feelings, and sensations in your body and behavior that you notice when you're too stressed.

The signs vary for different people. For me, I feel a slight twitch in my eyelid, I don't feel like talking to my friends, I have a tension in my shoulders, and I get irritated by the slightest disturbance. I'm reluctant to talk to others. What are your signs? Look back at Chapter 5 to remind yourself.

Step B: Breath and Beliefs

Breath

Take a few slow, deep mindful breaths. Then allow your breathing to be as it is and feel its sensation. Expand your awareness to your body and feel all the sensations there, accepting them as they are. Recognize any tight or tense bodily sensations as part and parcel of the stress response if that's what they are. No need to try to change the sensation—just watch and, if you can, accept them.

Beliefs

Now ask yourself: "What exactly am I stressed about?" Your answer may be "I'm concerned that I won't finish the report on time" or "I'm worried I'll run out of money this month." Then consider reevaluating your current beliefs about stress itself. It's not always easy, but see if you can give it a go. Think, "This stress is energizing me to prepare to complete the report" rather than just "I must reduce my stress" or "Stress is bad." Remember that stress can be healthy in short bursts as it sharpens your senses, strengthens you to act, releases oxytocin to urge you to be with others, and initially boosts your immune function. You could also reevaluate your stressor—for example, "Yes, I'm scared about running out of money for rent, but I could always borrow from Dad if worse comes to worst."

Step C: Choose a Mindful Action

This step is about choosing what to do next.

Whatever the stressor, you either need to change the situation or accept what you can't change.

If you decide that you need to change the situation: Maybe you need to call the employment agency, finish that report, or take your child home if he's having a tantrum.

If you decide you need to accept the situation, at least for now, you can:

- *Choose to do something energizing.* Consider going for a walk, run, jog, running up or down the stairs. The activity may help to burn up your stress hormones, which is what your body is gearing up to do—act. Integrate your activity with mindful awareness rather than just letting your mind worry.
- *Choose to do something relaxing.* This can be any activity that you have time for and that appeals to you. Here are some examples: have a bath, listen to music, garden, go for a drive, meditation, or yoga. Do the activity with mindful awareness.
- *Choose to be mindful in the moment.* You may choose just to be fully mindful in whatever you do next. This may be the case if you're traveling or at work or in the middle of a conversation. Just choose one of your senses and fully connect with it. Immerse your attention in the experience. Ideally, I'd recommend you be mindfully aware and have a spirit of kindness to yourself no matter which choice you make.

Reflection

Make a summary of the Mindful ABC Exercise if it appeals to you. When you try it out, write down what effect the exercise had on your state of mind, your emotions, and whether you dealt with the stressor differently from how you may normally have coped with it.

Raising Well-Being to Reduce Stress

If you're feeling even slightly distressed with the pressures of life, you're probably not feeling happy. You may not even believe that happiness is something achievable for you given your circumstances. And yet taking steps to raise your long-term well-being can increase your resilience to stress.

Researchers at the Harvard School of Public Health examined 200 studies on well-being and cardiovascular health. They found both positive emotion and optimism to slow the progression of heart disease and halve the risk of a major issue with your heart, such as a heart attack. So being happy both opens your emotional heart and heals your physical heart!

A fantastic model that I've been using to raise well-being in recent years is called the Five Ways to Well-Being. This is an evidence-based plan from the New Economics Foundation in the United Kingdom, based on the U.K. government's state-of-the-art research on mental well-being. Everyone's path to a life of happiness is different, but these activities have been found by research to be particularly beneficial for raising people's well-being and reduce distress.

The five ways to well-being, depicted in the diagram below, are:

1. **Connect**—This is about increasing the quality of your relationships with friends, family, coworkers, or even neighbors.
2. **Move**—This area emphasizes the importance of moving your body rather than being sedentary.
3. **Notice**—This is almost directly about mindfulness and how your awareness of your inner thoughts and emotions helps to clarify your values and direction in life. You also notice and appreciate the world around you.
4. **Discover**—This is about learning new things. Not necessarily through just books or courses or by earning certificates, but anything new.

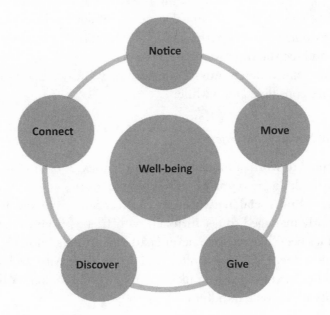

5. **Give**—This is about learning to give of yourself a little bit every day and enjoy the feeling of helping others. This too can help to enhance your connections and build the quality and depth of your social network.

A very small action in any one of these areas often has a lasting impact, just as a small pebble creates ripples throughout a lake. By improving one area, you'll start to improve them all. And, as you'll note in the descriptions that follow, mindfulness underlies them all.

CONNECT WITH OTHERS

A powerful way of raising your resilience to stress and enjoy greater well-being is through social relationships. Close relationships with family and friends offer love and support. Broader connections bring a sense of belonging. Seek to be close enough to a few people so you can turn to one another at times of difficulty.

> "I didn't notice any changes from practicing mindfulness, but my wife has! She says I'm much less reactive and nicer to be with. And when she says something like that, she means it! I can see it's improving our connection."

One of the great advantages of a conversation with someone you trust, when you're distressed, is putting things into perspective. As you'll recall, one of the core factors that drives stress is how you interpret the situation. If you're in an anxious state, that interpretation is not happening through the wise, calm part of your brain: the prefrontal cortex. Instead, it's a reaction arising from activation in the amygdala, the part that wants you to focus on danger and see the negative consequences.

Here are some different ways for developing your social network that you may not have considered for a while:

Ways of Making New Friends

- **Carpool to work.** Your employer may organize it, or just ask colleagues at work. It's a great way to get to know someone.
- **Use online social networks** to connect with your old friends. I've recently managed to get in touch with friends from primary school, and it's been like we were never apart when we met up.
- **Walk a dog.** Dog owners often end up chatting with each other. You could even volunteer to walk dogs from a local shelter. A nice opportunity to do some mindful walking too.

Ways of Deepening Your Current Relationships

- **Remember the golden rule:** Treat others the way you'd appreciate being treated yourself.
- **Invest time and energy in your close relationships.** That's the best investment you can make.
- **Give relationships some space.** Balance time together with time pursuing your own interests.
- **Be forgiving.** Everyone makes mistakes; we're all human.

Reflection

Write down who is closest to you in your life. Examples may include family, friends, colleagues, neighbors, mentors, and others.

You don't need to have lots of relationships. Even a small number of close relationships to people you can turn to in times of difficulty is fine. But if it's just one person, consider exploring ways to develop more close relationships with family or friends.

BE PHYSICALLY ACTIVE

Want to reduce your stress and increase your productivity? At the same time, want to reduce your risk of heart disease, stroke, and cancer by 50%? Then exercise is for you!

Any activity that doesn't involve passively sitting or lying down is a step in the right direction. Going to the gym is not the only way to be physically active. Find activities you enjoy and that are right for your current ability. And if you can do that exercise with others, even better.

Examples of exercise include:

- Walking briskly
- Playing tennis
- Pushing a lawn mower
- Using a vacuum cleaner

If the activity enables you to break a sweat, you're making your heart work and achieving benefits for your body and mind. Be creative and see what activities you can find that get you sweating!

When you combine these activities with mindfulness, the benefits are not just a physical release of tension, but a brain exercise too—staying in the present moment nonjudgmentally while your body moves. If you do your best to be mindful while doing the physical exercise, you're effectively meditating with all the extra benefits that brings.

How much activity should you do? That's a common question, and the best way for me to answer is to ask: How much activity are you willing to do? Even a 5-minute walk up and down your street has been found to have benefits. And there's mounting evidence that short bouts of exercise, like a brisk walk, can build fitness and help you manage stress.

If you don't do any physical activity at the moment, try these tips to get you moving.

- **Ask yourself:** Are you willing to give physical activity a try if it's fun? Physical activity will make you feel happier, healthier, and live longer. It will improve your brain function, make you feel more confident, help reduce smoking, and even lower your credit card bill, as you're less likely to spend money to feel better!
- **Boost your willpower.** You can do this by one of the following: getting to bed on time, practicing meditation, and eating foods with a low glycemic index (GI). Foods with a low GI are generally better for you, as they raise your blood sugar level slowly. With greater willpower, you'll be more likely to create an exercise habit.
- **Spend time with people who do exercise regularly.** You are more likely to think of physical activity positively if you have friends who do the same. They may inspire you to get moving.
- **Make a plan and measure.** By making a basic activity plan and recording what you achieved, you'll be much more likely to stick to it. You could use an app on your phone or simply record it in your journal or other notebook. Set a small, manageable goal to start with, like a 5-minute walk every day.
- **Be self-compassionate when you lapse.** On the days you don't manage to exercise, practice self-kindness. This is hard to believe for many people, but being too strict with yourself when you fail makes it more likely you'll fail again. Forgiving yourself puts you in a more positive mind-set, making another setback less likely.
- **Exercise with a friend.** If you can, find someone else to do your physical activities with. You can then motivate each other, and on the days you want to give up, your friend will encourage you.
- **Reduce your sitting time.** Even if you do half an hour of exercise a day, recent research has found if you spend hours at work sitting, the exercise makes a limited difference health-wise. Try standing while on

the phone, having a walking meeting, or going for a stroll at lunchtime. Stand and move throughout the day as much as you can.

TAKE NOTICE

Noticing or, in other words, mindfulness, helps you stimulate curiosity and appreciate the world around you. Rather than seeing life in a habitual way, you wake up and enjoy what's going well in your life. Connect with sights, sounds, smells, tastes, and touch. Noticing your own thoughts and feelings can also clarify what direction you want to go in life. So you're making conscious decisions, not being set in your old ways.

Apart from practicing meditation, yoga, or tai chi, here are some more unusual ways of improving your noticing skills:

- **Watch for all objects with a certain color** for a few minutes. For example, if I pick green, I can now notice trees, grass, a highlighter pen, a logo on a business card, a part of my teacup, and a pattern on my curtain.
- **Do one task at half the normal speed for just 1 minute.** What else do you then notice? If I try that while typing, I suddenly notice how smooth the keys are and that I'm sitting in a twisted posture.
- **Try doing nothing for 5 minutes a day.** Yup, nothing. Just sit there or lie there and see what happens. If that's really difficult to do, due to time pressure, maybe you need to look at managing your time differently.
- **Count how many different sounds you can hear when you're waiting in a queue.** When I stop to try this, I notice cars in the distance, a boiling kettle, a distant plane, and plates being clattered. I wasn't aware of any of that before.
- **Ask yourself three questions:** How do I feel right now? What am I thinking about right now? What can I notice with my senses right now?

DISCOVER

Learning something new raises your confidence. And because whatever you're learning is new, you naturally become more mindful in the process. Imagine learning to paint or drive for the first time—your attention would be fully in the present as you develop the new skill.

Most people associate learning with school. But your brain is built and thrives on learning new things, and you can learn at any age. And when you learn by doing activities, that learning is enhanced.

Here are some ideas for ways you can keep learning to build resilience and mental well-being:

- Ask the people around you more questions.
- Seek to learn one new fact every day.
- Take a course in painting, playing an instrument, or fixing cars.
- Engage in a new role at work.
- Try playing a new sport, listening to a new audiobook, or cooking something different.
- Visit a museum to learn about a period you find interesting in history, art, or science.
- Try that hobby you've been thinking about, whether it's flying toy helicopters, knitting, or writing fiction.

I've recently tried painting. I must say, I had ideas like "I can't paint!" running through my head the first time. But splashing colors on a canvas and making mistakes was highly therapeutic and fun. I just called it modern art. I've been experimenting with meditating before doing the painting to see what effect that has—it made the paintings more serene and calming to look at. Other things I do to boost learning: listen to a new audiobook every couple of weeks, watch talks on *www.ted.com*, visit museums when I can, read blogs on science and psychology, read new books and go to lectures and talks on different topics from time to time.

GIVE

You may be surprised to see giving as a recommendation in a chapter on taking care of yourself. But both small and large acts of kindness can boost your sense of well-being, improve your relationships, and help you manage stress in a positive way. Being kind to others is an act of kindness to yourself. Kind people live longer and happier lives. People over age 55 who volunteer for two or more organizations have a 44% lower chance of dying. That's more effective than exercising four times a week!

I discovered a powerful example of this last week. An old friend visited me. After failing several years at university, becoming stressed and frustrated, he visited his doctor, who diagnosed him with chronic fatigue syndrome (CFS). His doctor advised him to find the time to help others rather than just rest. This seems like strange advice to someone who struggles to have the energy to do his own daily chores. But he took the advice and volunteered for a CFS charity. He began to feel grateful for what he could do, and helping others gave his life meaning again. He now also meditates and is far more positive and upbeat about his future. He enjoys the challenges in his life rather than feeling crushed by the stress. It seems that giving of himself has helped him reduce stress and increase his happiness.

Here are some ways you can give:

- Praise a colleague with a short e-mail.
- Open the door for someone.
- Make a cup of tea for a coworker.
- Smile more.
- Consider volunteering for the local community.
- Offer to help an elderly person with his or her bag.
- Invite a friend for dinner.
- Offer to help a colleague with a work project.

> "I love the feeling of doing something nice for someone else. That was one of my favorite parts of Shamash's course for me. It gave me permission to be nice just for the sake of itself. It lifted my mood every time! It's amazing that I rarely made time to do this before."

EXERCISE: Improving One Area of Your Lifestyle

If you feel overwhelmed with all the things that could improve your well-being, stress not! Try the following steps to clarify one action you could do. Just one action is a fine way to start.

1. Look at the diagram of the five ways to well-being on page 247. Rate how well you're doing in each area on a scale of 1 to 5: 1 for lots of potential for improvement in that area and 5 for doing perfectly well in that area of your life right now, in your opinion.
2. Decide which area you want to develop. You may choose the lowest-value one or the one that you'd most like to develop. It's better to choose the area you're most likely to be successful in and would enjoy.
3. In this coming week, take action in the area you've chosen. For example, if it's Discover, see what new things you learn every day already. Perhaps play a new game with your child, rediscover an old hobby, or join that evening class you've been meaning to take.
4. Do your tiny chosen activity in a mindful way. Savor the experience. And watch to see if you begin to cope better with your

stress. Finish by recording your findings in your journal. And if you're inspired, take another action next month!

Measure to Motivate Yourself

Measuring your daily activities is a great way to boost your motivation. You can measure not only how much exercise you do but also your heart rate, the quality of your sleep, your weight, your mood, how you use your time, the amount of meditation you've done, the number of steps you've taken in a day, and more. Recently my mother started using a pedometer to record how many steps she takes a day, and it has helped motivate her to walk more.

There is now a whole movement based on measuring yourself to help you achieve your goals. It's called quantified self, and you can start exploring at *www.quantifiedself.com*.

I'm into technology and for the last few months have used a variety of applications on my phone to keep track, which is motivating for me and has helped me develop healthy habits. I've been tracking the amount of time I spend meditating (insight meditation timer app), my weight and eating habits (My Fitness Pal app), the number of walks or runs I do every week and my speed (Runkeeper app), how I use my time (just on Excel), and the quality of my sleep (Sleep Cycle app) and recording my thoughts in my own journal, which I do privately online (*www.penzu.com*). If you don't like using technology, you can simply keep records using a pen and paper—that's just as good and perhaps less stressful for you!

PRACTICE: Mindful Yoga and Meditation for Life

 10 minutes.

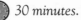 *30 minutes.*

By now, you're familiar with the yoga sequences that have been offered to you. Today you're invited to practice in silence and to start the practice with a 5-minute standing body scan. You can use this body scan to find out which areas of your body are tense and require some attention, and which areas are relaxed. Then engage in whatever yoga postures you feel your body needs. Rather than thinking of the yoga practice as something unusual that you do, allow the yoga stretches to feel like a natural process. Just as you naturally stretch your body in the morning in bed, stretch your body with mindful awareness to meet your body's current needs.

After practicing this for 10 or 30 minutes, depending on whether you're doing the mini or full course, go on to practice any mindfulness meditation of your choice. Again, try doing this without using the audio.

VARIATION: Just for a change, you could try practicing the meditation first and then doing the yoga. Notice what effect that has. Your level of mindful awareness in the yoga may increase.

The Daffodils

I wandered lonely as a cloud
That floats on high o'er vales and hills,
When all at once I saw a crowd,
A host, of golden daffodils;
Beside the lake, beneath the trees,
Fluttering and dancing in the breeze.

Continuous as the stars that shine
And twinkle on the milky way,
They stretched in never-ending line
Along the margin of a bay:
The thousand saw I at a glance,
Tossing their heads in sprightly dance.

The waves beside them danced; but they
Outdid the sparkling waves in glee:
A poet could not but be gay,
In such a jocund company:
I gazed—and gazed—but little thought
What wealth the show to me had brought:

For oft, when on my couch I lie
In vacant or in pensive mood,
They flash upon that inward eye
Which is the bliss of solitude;
And then my heart with pleasure fills,
And dances with the daffodils.
                    —WILLIAM WORDSWORTH

Reflection: How Was Your Day of Mindfulness?

If you chose to have a day, or perhaps half-day, of mindfulness, how did you find the experience? What did you like or not like about it? What did you discover about your thoughts, emotions, bodily sensations, urges, and desires? If you plan to have another such day, do you wish to pop the date in your diary, or just see when it feels right?

Record your reflections in your journal, phone, or tablet.

Self-Care FAQs

Q: **I'm already doing things for others all the time. Are you really suggesting I give more of myself?**

A: If you're already giving your time to help others, you don't have to give any more. For you, perhaps you need to give less by saying no more often. But many people spend their time thinking about themselves and their own lives to feel better when actually seeking to help others would help themselves. This is because the brain is hardwired to reward you when you're generous with your time or energy. As the Dalai Lama says, "If you want others to be happy, practice compassion. If you want to be happy, practice compassion."

Q: **I literally have no spare time for mindfulness with my young baby and job. I'm on the go from morning till I fall asleep exhausted. What can I do?**

A: If you have no spare slots to stop and practice a mindfulness exercise like the mindful pause, then don't worry! You can practice mindfulness as you are doing your daily activities. When you're looking at your child, pay attention to her eyes and body and gently smile at her rather than letting your mind get too lost in planning and worrying. When breastfeeding, be there with your child. When driving to the doctor for a checkup, feel your breath and notice the world around you, ensuring you switch off your phone and other distractions. Micro moments of mindfulness make a difference—a deep breath here, a mindful hug there—it all makes a huge difference.

Q: **I'm anxious about this course ending. How can I prepare for the end?**

A: This course isn't the end, really. If anything, it's the beginning of a journey into a life of greater mindfulness. Seek to join a local mindfulness or meditation group in your area, and if there isn't one, consider an online mindfulness group, either mine or some other one that appeals. Perhaps in the near future, you can start a mindfulness group of your own to support others as well as yourself in the practice.

Q: I love the loving-kindness meditation! Can I just do that one?

A: Yes, you can! You can do any meditation you like. Different people like different meditations. They have all been found to be beneficial, so use what works for you or whatever you enjoy.

Q: Unfortunately, I never really got into the mindfulness practice in this book. I'm not good at sticking to things like this. What shall I do?

A: That's okay—you're not alone! There are two approaches you could take. You could closely watch your thoughts and find out what ideas you have that are preventing you from practicing the mindful experiments. And then begin by fully committing to doing 1 minute of meditation every day and building up from there. Alternatively, consider what hobbies or physical activity you do regularly and make that activity a mindful one. Even if it's knitting mindfully three or four times a week, that would be great.

Home Experiments: Week 7

This week, experiment with not using the guided audio when you meditate. Instead, just set a timer for however long you choose to meditate. And you can choose whatever meditation you prefer or feel would work best for you. If you find practicing without the audio too difficult, then try using the audio on alternate days.

Mindful Booster

This week, the mindful booster is to use the ABC approach to stress that you discovered in this chapter. To summarize it, A is awareness, so become aware of your stress signs, including thoughts, feelings, body, and behavior. Step B is about becoming aware of your breath and then also becoming aware of your beliefs about stress and shifting your thoughts to a more positive attitude toward the stress itself.

See your beating heart as strengthening you. Feel a faster breathing rate as oxygenating your brain and body. Finally, step C is choice. Choose a relaxing activity to lower stress to more manageable levels; or an energizing activity to channel your vitality; or face your stressor and try to fix things so your stress is effectively managed. Work with your stress rather than just trying to eliminate or run away from it.

Week 7

Day	Mini-Course	Full Course
1	Any mini-meditation you like, without audio Mindful booster: Try the ABC approach to stress	Any full meditation practice you like, without audio Mindful pause × 3 Mindful booster: Try the ABC approach to stress
2	Any mini-meditation you like, without audio Mindful booster: Try the ABC approach to stress	Any full meditation practice you like, without audio Mindful pause × 3 Mindful booster: Try the ABC approach to stress
3	Any mini-meditation you like, without audio Mindful booster: Try the ABC approach to stress	Any full meditation practice you like, without audio Mindful pause × 3 Mindful booster: Try the ABC approach to stress
4	Any mini-meditation you like, without audio Mindful booster: Try the ABC approach to stress	Any full meditation practice you like, without audio Mindful pause × 3 Mindful booster: Try the ABC approach to stress
5	Any mini-meditation you like, without audio Mindful booster: Try the ABC approach to stress	Any full meditation practice you like, without audio Mindful pause × 3 Mindful booster: Try the ABC approach to stress
6	Any mini-meditation you like, without audio Mindful booster: Try the ABC approach to stress	Any full meditation practice you like, without audio Mindful pause × 3 Mindful booster: Try the ABC approach to stress

TWELVE

Week 8

The Rest of Your Life

*You have brains in your head. You have feet in your
shoes. You can steer yourself any direction you choose.
You're on your own. And you know what you know.
And YOU are the one who'll decide where to go. . . .*

—Dr. Seuss

INTENTIONS

+ *To reflect on what you discovered in this course.*

+ *To look at how you now handle acute stress having done this course.*

+ *To explore how to continue practicing mindfulness.*

+ *To set your vision for a more mindful life with clear intentions for both the
short and long term.*

RAJ WAS a single man in his late 30s. He worked as a dentist in a busy
local practice. He'd divorced a year earlier after being married for about
a year. It goes without saying, but his ex had seemed so wonderful when
they were dating—the perfect lady. After they got married, alarm bells
immediately started to ring. Her expectations of him increased dramatically, and they argued every night. No matter what he tried to improve
the relationship, she just kept demanding more of him. After 12 months
of agony, stress, and misery, they ended the relationship.

After the stress of divorce, life began to settle down again. His stress
levels were slowly beginning to return to normal. Except for one thing.
Raj had started spending money to make himself feel better through the

divorce, and the habit hadn't stopped. He just couldn't stop spending money. Designer clothes that he just *had* to have. Holidays at luxurious hotels. All the latest gadgets. He bought a new car, thinking he "deserved it." Finally, he even got a mortgage on a house that he couldn't afford. Most evenings were spent surfing the Web and making new purchases. Eventually, he stopped opening bills that dropped through the mail slot every day, and before he knew it, he'd maxed out his credit cards.

When a colleague said they were going to come to one of my mindfulness classes, he decided to give it a try—he'd read about mindfulness in a magazine. Raj discovered his body was riddled with tension, and the body scan meditation started to release that naturally. He meditated every day and with each session, worked through a whole host of emotions that he'd pushed away over the last couple of years.

The meditations started to clear his mind. He began to feel confident enough to open the bills and make the necessary phone calls. He also started to take better care of his health, jogging occasionally in the mornings and preparing healthy meals for himself a few days a week.

But the best thing for him was that he stopped overspending. He realized he kept purchasing online to feel the euphoria of having a new gadget, shirt, or laptop. But that feeling didn't last long. Within about 15 minutes, the desire to buy one more thing arose. He was then shopping again to recreate that excitement. The next time he felt the urge to shop, he hesitated. He did a mindful pause and noticed the sense of desire as a tangible body sensation. He then set a timer for 5 minutes to see whether he could feel the urge together with his breath to see what happens. He managed. But amazingly, the urge had passed within about 2 minutes.

That autopilot behavior to shop began to drop away, replaced by meditation practice. The mindfulness organically grew a sense of deep-seated well-being in his heart. No amount of shopping could offer him that same inner peace.

PRACTICE: Coming Full Circle

Before you dive into this week's session, start with some mindfulness meditation practice, as outlined below. The meditations will help you have a more mindful outlook for the reflections that follow in the session.

Body Scan

⏱ *10 minutes.*

⏱ *30 minutes.*

Audio tracks 6 and 7.

You started this mindfulness course with the body scan meditation, lying down and taking up to half an hour to get in touch with the sensations in your body from moment to moment. We now come full circle.

When you first tried the body scan, you may have experienced a whole host of different ideas, opinions, and beliefs about what to expect. After almost 2 months of mindfulness practice, you can bring a different quality to the experience today.

In particular, try bringing the following two attitudes to your body scan:

1. **Acceptance.** Notice whether your mind just keeps wandering relentlessly. See if you can accept that. Notice whether you feel pain, discomfort, or a sense of wanting to move, fidget, or relax. See if you can accept that. Notice any emotions that arise through your practice of the body scan and see if you can accept that too. Give the space for all experiences to just be, rather than trying to change them. Smile at thoughts like "but I've been meditating for 2 months and I still can't control my mind" and just start again. Remember, we're not in the business of *controlling* thoughts.

2. **Freshness.** By this I mean experiencing as if for the very first time. Sometimes this is called practicing with "beginner's mind." Practice the body scan as if you've never done the body scan before, with a sense of curiosity and openness.

I know for me personally, the body scan is more challenging than the sitting meditation as I'm more prone to fall asleep, but even so, I find I become more in tune with my bodily sensations throughout the day after the meditation.

Yoga Stretches

10 minutes.

30 minutes.

Audio tracks 9 and 10 (optional).

Following the body scan, practice some mindful yoga or mindful stretching of your choice. You can use a guided audio or simply tune in to your own bodily sensations to decide which body parts need stretching. Continue to bring the attitudes of acceptance and beginner's mind, as you did in the body scan.

Expanding Awareness Meditation

⏱ *Audio tracks 15 and 16 (optional).*

⏱ Finally, after the yoga, spend some time in this meditation. This is usually practiced in a seated posture. Again, use a guided audio of your choice, or simply set a timer for however long you wish. Notice how it feels to do the meditation after the body scan and yoga practice. Do you find the experience easier or more challenging?

Reflection

Write down what your experience of the meditations was like today.

1. Did you manage to bring a little more acceptance or beginner's mind?
2. Was it a struggle? Was there something you were not accepting? If so, what?
3. Was there any aspect of the meditation you enjoyed?
4. Do you find yourself judging the practice as "a good session" or "a bad one"? If so, how could you describe it differently?

Reflecting on the Course: What Gems Did You Discover?

At this point, it's useful to reflect on what you've discovered about yourself by reading this book and practicing the meditations. Some insights may have come from simply reading the words on this page. Others, through the actual experience of meditation. Or you may have made a discovery when being mindful in your everyday life.

These insights are important. By taking some time to look back over the course and reflecting on your insights, you can grow in wisdom and self-understanding.

For example, when I first did a mindfulness course, my major insight about myself was this: Thoughts are just thoughts popping into my head; I don't always have to believe them or act on them. Also, I discovered that rather than spending every minute thinking, it's helpful to live in the moment and enjoy life just as it is.

Okay, now it's your turn!

EXERCISE: Self-Reflection Meditation

Take 10–15 minutes to do this meditation before entering reflections in your journal.

1. Start with a few minutes of mindfulness of breath.

2. Once you feel you've settled into the meditation, cast your mind back to the start of this meditation course. What did you discover when doing the eating meditation and the body scan?

3. You also explored the expanding awareness meditation, yoga, and the mindful pause. What did you enjoy about them? What did you discover from them?

4. As you went through the course, you learned about stress—both its benefits and its drawbacks. How has your understanding of stress developed?

5. Being as honest with yourself as you can, consider the following question: What are the most important insights you've discovered from this course that you wish to take away with you?

Reflection

Write down your answers to the questions asked in the preceding meditation, especially the last question.

Tales of Wisdom: Three Hairs

Once upon a time there was a woman who woke up, looked in the mirror, and noticed she had only three hairs on her head. She thought, "Oh well, I think I'll braid my hair today." She did so and had a great day.

The next day, she woke up, looked in the mirror, and found only two hairs on her head. "Hmmm," she thought. "I know—I'll part my hair down the middle today." And off she went and had a great day.

The next morning, she woke, looked in the mirror, and found just one hair on her head. "Oh . . . I can wear my hair just like a ponytail," she thought and, with a spring in her step, had a lovely day.

Waking up the next morning, she looked in the mirror and discovered she had no hair on her head at all. "Yay, I don't have to fix my hair today!" she thought.

Week 8 Is the Rest of Your Life!

Although this is the last session, I hope it's the beginning of a lifetime of mindfulness practice for you. This chapter will not only explore your next steps for this week but also create a realistic and exciting vision for the long term.

Some people want to just be mindful in their everyday life, without stopping to meditate even for a few minutes. That sounds great in theory, but in practice your mind easily goes back to its habitual ways. So if you're eager to be a more mindful person, you'll need to practice some meditation on a daily basis.

If you're suffering from chronic stress, practice as much mindfulness meditation as you can. The research shows the more you practice, the better it is for you. Monks who have been practicing all their lives have brains highly wired for resilience to stress according to brain scans. The half-hour body scans, expanding awareness meditations, and yoga may be best suited for your needs, which were part of the full program in this book.

If your challenge is short bursts of high stress (acute stress), then you need to use mindfulness to both respond to that stress effectively and find rest between those high-stress periods. A combination of mini-meditations when you're under pressure and the longer meditations from time to time may serve your purposes well.

"Before this course, I saw stress as the enemy. Now I understand that stress has evolved to help me. I use mindfulness to work with my stress, not against it."

If, having done this course, you just don't think meditation is for you, then consider doing one daily, solitary activity in a mindful way. Many people find running a mindful activity—time to de-stress and live in the now. For others it's walking the dog every morning, knitting, playing an instrument, cooking, or gardening. Find out what works for you and try to do it daily or as close to daily as you can.

Whatever you decide for your future, I hope the exercises that follow will help you clarify and stick to your chosen mindfulness practices so they help manage your stress. And when you aren't able to stick to your plan, remember to use mindfulness, curiosity, and self-kindness to gently get back on track, rather than creating another stressor in your life.

Setting Your Vision

Martin Luther King's famous "I Have a Dream" speech is considered one of the greatest orations of all time. It was particularly moving because King used imagery to set a vision of how he saw the future. And that dream, that vision, became a burning desire in people's hearts, moving them to action to make the vision a reality. Change began through imagery first and then action.

Einstein also understood the importance of imagination. He famously said, "Imagination is more important than knowledge." This statement seems strange coming from someone who is considered so knowledgeable. But as you may know, one of Einstein's greatest ideas came through his imagining what it would be like to ride on a beam of light.

Today you have the chance to use your own imagination to create a vision for your future mindful self. A vision of how you'll be using mindfulness in your life to work with stress. This may seem ironic, as mindfulness emphasizes living in the present. But when you have a powerful yet attainable vision, you are more highly motivated to take action in the present.

You'll do this in several stages, shown in the diagram on page 266:

1. Create a long-term vision through a letter-writing exercise and then come up with three long-term goals you're excited about.
2. Create a short-term vision through a reflection exercise and then come up with three short-term goals you're excited about.
3. Decide on a meditation schedule based on your previous reflections and visions if that's what you wish.
4. Through the daily meditations and your efforts to live in the present moment, you're living with greater levels of mindful awareness, helping you work with stress more creatively.

YOUR LONG-TERM VISION

Recent research has found that if people don't imagine or feel a connection with their future self, they are much less likely to eat healthily or exercise. One piece of research found that people who felt as if their future self was like

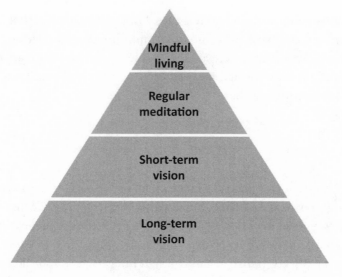

some other person, rather than themselves, took less care of themselves and even saved less for retirement!

If you develop a closer connection to your future self, you will be more likely to keep to your goal of regular mindfulness meditation or other daily mindful practice. The following exercise has been tested on others and helps with this.

EXERCISE: Writing a Letter from Your Future Self

Imagine yourself at some future date. A year, 3 years, or perhaps even 10 years from now—whatever feels right to you. At this time, imagine you've learned to respond to your stress in a positive way. Imagine yourself as your ideal, future self, living with mindfulness, wisdom, compassion, or any other values that you consider important for you.

Visualize what it feels like to be a regular meditator if that's what you want. What time of day do you meditate? Where do you do your regular meditation practice? How willing are you to meditate when obstacles get in the way? When time is short? When stress levels are high?

Also consider how you respond to your everyday challenges. What's your response when stuck in traffic? How do you communicate with your partner, your friends, or your colleagues at work? How do you deal with conflicts? How mindful are you when you eat, when you exercise, and when you work? How aware are you of your moment-to-moment thoughts, feelings, and bodily sensations?

When you're ready, imagine that you, as your future self, can write to you as your present self. Write to your present self with the following points:

- Tell your present self all your **good qualities** that your future self can see. Explain to your present self all the strengths and skills you have that will make you more mindful and effective under pressure.
- Let your future self express **appreciation** for all the effort that your present self made to meditate regularly, practicing mindful walking, or whatever else you wish to do.
- Offer your present self some **self-compassionate words of wisdom** to overcome your present challenges in being mindful and dealing with your stress.

Here's an excerpt from a letter that I wrote a few years back to my present self when going through some tough challenges at work and wanting to be a writer and meditation teacher.

Dear Present-Day Shamash,

How are you? I hope you're well. It's your future self, Shamash, here! I'm writing to encourage you to gently stick with your mindfulness practice to deal with the stress you're currently facing.

Good qualities

I know things seem difficult for you at the moment with all the challenges at work. But you have great strengths to get you through them. You're creative and come up with unique solutions to the challenges you face. You're willing to put the effort in to find solutions rather than just give up. You love mindfulness and by practicing meditation every day you'll be better able to handle the stress that comes your way. And on the days you don't meditate, you can forgive yourself—you never need to be hard on yourself.

Appreciation

I know you're going through a tough time at the moment, with all the classes you teach, the prep you have to do, some aggressive managers and personal issues. But I'm writing to say a big thank-you for sticking with the meditation and mindful practice. Doing regular days and half-days of mindfulness practice really helped you. You worked hard to get through this tough time and became a more stress-resilient person for doing so.

Self-compassionate words of wisdom

You're going through a tough time at the moment, but you're not alone. It's not such a big deal in the great scheme of things. So many people are faced with difficult challenges at work. No need to be hard on yourself. Instead, say nice things to yourself, like, "Hey, you tried your best," or "Today was tough, but tomorrow is another day." These words of self-kindness may feel strange, but they are exactly what you'd say to a friend going through difficulties. Over the years it will become second nature to you.

In conclusion, thanks once again for persevering with the daily meditation and mindful living and for being compassionate to both yourself and others. And remember, the challenges you're facing are temporary—they will pass. Be mindful!

Love,
Future Shamash

(TIPS) Write in your own style—there's no need for you to copy me in any way. Feel free to add extra sections, and you can write in much more detail.

Take your time with this exercise. You may like to do it after practicing a meditation.

If letter writing doesn't inspire you, consider a painting, collage, or whatever other form of expression works for you.

Reflection

Following your letter, you should have some ideas for three realistic, long-term goals for living a more mindful life to manage your stress. Write them down.

Examples include practicing mindfulness meditation for 15 minutes a day, doing a day of mindfulness every few months, doing a mindfulness course annually, cultivating friendships through mindful communication, or whatever else you would like to see yourself doing in a mindful way.

YOUR SHORT-TERM INTENTIONS: THE NEXT 3 MONTHS

You've been practicing mindfulness for about 2 months now. For some of you, meditation may have become a daily habit. Others may have struggled to find the time and space to meditate regularly and perhaps feel frustrated about that.

Having considered your long-term vision, think about what goals related to mindfulness to manage your stress you'd like to achieve over the next 3 months. One of your goals may be a daily meditation practice, one could be about living in a mindful way or applying one of the mindful boosters, and one goal could be to go for a mindful walk for 15 minutes every day. To help you clarify your goals and increase your chances of success rather than making the goals into another source of stress, try writing down the specifics of your plan.

> "My vision is to be a peaceful, happy person—someone who looks after himself. In the last 8 weeks, this dream is becoming a reality. It's much closer than I thought."

Reflection

Write down your mindfulness plan for the next 3 months. Answer the following questions to improve your chances of building a mindfulness habit:

1. What are your three main goals or intentions for the next 3 months? It's important to be as realistic as you can.
2. Which meditations will you do each month?
3. How much time will you spend doing them?
4. What time of day will you do them?
5. What are the chances that you're going to stick to this plan?
6. Is there any way of increasing your chances? If so, how?
7. Who can you talk to about this plan, to improve your chances of success? Or is there someone you could meditate with on a daily or weekly basis?
8. What are all the obstacles that will prevent you from doing your meditation practice? Be as honest with yourself as you can.
9. When these obstacles arise, what action could you realistically take to help overcome them?
10. What words of kindness could you use at the times when you don't achieve your goal (treating yourself like you would a good friend)?

Reflecting on obstacles is particularly important. Most people think the best way to stick to your goals is to think positively about them. But it

Research Corner: Achieving Your Intentions

To explain why setting your intentions and writing them all down is so important, consider the following study published in the *British Journal of Health Psychology* in 2010. Researchers studied how best to help people stick to their goals by testing 248 people and put them randomly in three groups, hoping to get them to start exercising.

- Group 1—Control: They asked them to keep track of how much they exercised over 2 weeks.
- Group 2—Motivation: They asked them to read a leaflet all about the benefits of exercise to reduce heart disease. They were then told to track their exercise over the next 2 weeks.
- Group 3—Intention: This group received the same leaflet as Group 2. But they were also asked to write down, there and then, what day and time they would do their 20 minutes of vigorous exercise over the next week.

Here are the surprising results:

- Group 1: 38% exercised at least once a week.
- Group 2: 35% exercised at least once a week.
- Group 3: 91% exercised at least once a week!

This suggests, along with many other studies, that if you write down specifically when and where you are going to do your chosen activity (in our case, mindful living and meditation), you're much more likely to achieve your goal. It also suggests that just reading about the benefits of mindfulness to motivate yourself may not work on its own—you need to commit to dates and times and write them down.

---

turns out that it's even more effective to think negatively—to think about what might prevent you from achieving your goal and determining what you'll do to handle that.

For me the thought "Oh, I can't be bothered to meditate now" can be the obstacle to meditating if I'm feeling really tired or agitated. And if I go down for breakfast and start my day, I'm much less likely to meditate. So I watch out for that thought and desire and say to myself, "Let me meditate for at least 1 minute and then decide." Usually after the first minute, I'm happy to keep going. In fact, this technique works for me on other tasks I'm procrastinating over too!

Installing the Meditation Habit

To make mindfulness meditation a daily occurrence, you need to make it into a habit. This may seem strange, as you've discovered the problem of living in a habitual, autopilot way. But you can make the habit of meditation a conscious one, rather than doing it automatically. Conscious good habits are ones you are aware you have and are happy to have. The meditation habit is one such example.

I've made meditation a daily, morning habit. Most mornings I just get up and meditate. So I don't need to really think or debate or force myself too much. There have been some times when I've slipped out of the habit, but I've managed to reinstate the habit before too long. You can achieve a similar, positive habit.

There has been quite a lot of research on how to form good habits in recent years. Here's what the science suggests.

1. **Take small steps.** As you're new to meditation, the 30 minutes or even the 10 minutes a day may have been too tricky. If so, try 3 minutes a day—you decide what you can do and stick to it! You can then build from there.
2. **Focus on one habit at a time.** If you're creating a habit of daily meditation, don't also make major changes in other areas of your life, like eating or exercising habits. Focus on one change at a time to increase the likelihood of success. Many experiments have shown humans don't have unlimited willpower, so choosing your challenges one at a time is a great idea.
3. **Write your goal down.** Use your journal to record how much you want to meditate, what time you plan to do so, and by what date you wish to achieve this. You've already done this if you did the last journaling exercise.
4. **Repeat, repeat.** To form a habit to meditate, you need to keep practicing. How many times? It varies from person to person—you'll know meditation has become a habit when it becomes second nature.

Charles Duhigg, in his bestselling book *The Power of Habit*, identifies three parts of a neurological habit loop. They are simply:

1. Cue
2. Routine
3. Reward

In the case of meditation practice, the routine is the meditation practice itself. What's the cue? That's the trigger that tells your mind it's time to meditate. For me, the cue is simply waking up in the morning. After I wake up, I have a little natural stretch in bed, set my meditation timer or listen to a guided meditation, and meditate. Experiments show triggers can be in the following categories:

- **Location.** For example, one of my clients always meditates on the train to work. That's his cue to meditate.
- **Time.** Whatever particular time you choose. Mornings are often best, but not for everyone.
- **Emotion.** For example, you may meditate when you feel anxious, low, angry, or tired. These can be your meditation triggers.
- **Other people.** For example, you may meditate together with a friend or when you attend a meditation group.
- **Previous action.** For example, after brushing your teeth or after breakfast or after taking a shower.

So, what about the reward? In meditation, the idea is to simply practice and observe what arises rather than seeking a reward. I know that if I stop meditating for a week, I become more irritable, less calm, and less focused. Being a more accepting, peaceful, and focused person makes me feel better. That's my reward. Some teachers would say there's no reward to meditation; you practice for its own sake.

(TIP) When you're first creating your meditation habit, you could experiment with rewarding yourself with a call to a friend, your favorite meal, or a cup of your favorite coffee. A little reward after meditating will help create that habit loop in your brain. After a while, you no longer need to reward yourself with external things; the meditation itself will be your reward.

This Too Will Pass

When things get too much, you can take no more,
When getting out of bed seems the biggest chore.
There are four words that can give you peace,
No matter what the anxiety, it's sure to cease.
The words are simple, their meaning clear,
Remember them now, and hold them dear.
For all experiences are relatively brief,
Think "This too will pass" and smile with relief!
—SHAMASH ALIDINA

Mindfulness Is Miraculous but Takes Her Time

The Grand Canyon is considered one of the Seven Wonders of the World—a miracle of nature. Its immensity can almost overwhelm your senses. The canyon averages 4,000 feet in depth for over 277 miles! And that depth has been cut by the Colorado River. For the river to achieve this, it has taken millions of years. When I visited a few years ago, I couldn't even see the river at the bottom. And yet it was amazing how deep the canyon was. A reminder of what can be achieved over time.

In the same way, your daily practice of mindfulness may not seem to make any difference on a daily basis. You may feel frustrated that you continue to feel the rough bristles of excessive stress rub against you. But the river of awareness sinks deep in your being. Day by day, mindful awareness softens your heart and awakens your senses to the rich beauty of life around you. Just remember the Colorado River—each day the river cuts a fraction of a millimeter, but over time develops a world's wonder. But here's the good news: although meditation may take months to fully show its effects, it doesn't take millions of years like the Colorado River!

The pain of life can feel as if it leaves permanent scars within you. And yet the soft gentleness of mindfulness can begin healing those wounds within. You may feel broken, damaged, even beyond repair. You are not alone in these feelings. Mindfulness is not the answer to all your problems; it's one answer. But I've met so many people who have found mindfulness to be a soothing, healing solution to life's relentless stresses. They describe mindfulness as a lifesaver, a chance to start again.

For example, Lucy was a trainee accountant. She had lots of pressure at work and had to study for accountancy exams in the evenings. She had no time to see her friends. On top of this, her boss never seemed happy with any of her work. One day she randomly burst into tears—she felt so stressed. Within weeks, her boyfriend left her, saying she had no time for him. Her life felt like it was falling apart. Lucy couldn't face work anymore. She went to see her doctor, who gave her time off and recommended a mindfulness program. The meditations taught her to separate herself from her relentless waves of negative thoughts and feelings. This helped her start feeling in control of her life. The mindfulness taught her that self-acceptance was more important than trying to be perfect at work. She went for mindful walks in her local park and reconnected with her friends. Within a few months, she rejoined her company in a different department and went on to build a successful career. She continues to make time for mindfulness practice daily. Years later, she still discovers new insights about herself and others through her mindful and self-compassion exercises. The painful experience of anxiety and loss she felt scarred her on the inside, but the meditations gave her the time and space to heal herself. You too have this inner capacity to heal, and mindfulness is a powerful way to access that.

Seven Keys to Unlocking a Mindful Lifestyle

As we approach the end of this chapter and course, I'm going to offer some suggestions for living mindfully, based on the acronym MINDFUL to make it easier for you to remember. If you like it, photocopy or download and print the diagram (see next page) that summarizes these keys (available to download and print from *www.guilford.com/alidina-materials*) and stick it up on your fridge door or somewhere else to remind you to be mindful. Think of it as a summary of the whole course.

M—MEDITATE

Spend a few minutes feeling your breath to a full body scan, expanding awareness meditation, or yoga practice. Meditation means to pay attention to your thoughts, feeling, body, breath, or to connect with one of your senses for a length of time that you choose. Feel free to be creative in what you think of as your daily meditation practice. Drinking tea, swimming, or gardening can all become a meditation when you do them intentionally and with mindful attention in the present moment. Consider adding a small smile as you meditate to remind you not to take the exercise too seriously. This reminds you to be less serious and more playful in your approach.

I—INTERPRET DIFFERENTLY

Only 10% of your well-being is determined by your outer circumstances. Change your attitude, your interpretation of events, to live a better life. Losing a job sucks, but does it give you a chance to change careers? A tight deadline isn't fun, but will the stress help to energize and motivate you to work more efficiently? To take an extreme example, when my grandparents died, I was upset and sad, of course; I was very close to them. But as time went by I realized that their death also helped the rest of our family become closer. We had a chance to celebrate their life. Their death is sad but also a chance for us to use the gifts they gave us. Interpretation is about directing your attention to the positive, not just the negative.

Seven Keys to a Mindful Lifestyle

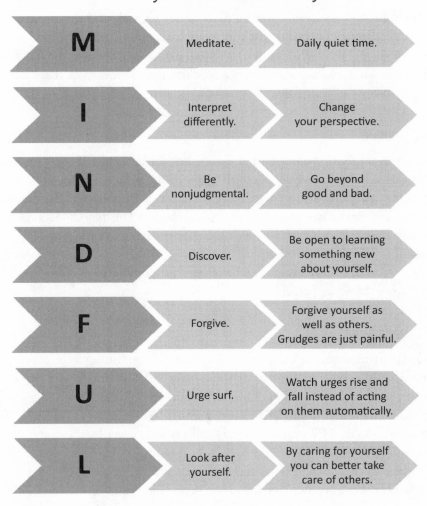

From *The Mindful Way through Stress*. Copyright 2015 by The Guilford Press.

N—BE NONJUDGMENTAL

When you're practicing mindfulness, the idea is to be nonjudgmental. Our perfectionistic society has trained us to perpetually look for what's wrong and try to improve it. But recall the last time you saw a scene of great beauty—perhaps a beautiful landscape of rolling hills and trees. Did you think, "That tree's a bit short" or "That hill isn't quite curvy enough"? Of course not. You looked nonjudgmentally. You were mindful and enjoyed the moment. You can judge to make decisions, but make time to stop judging every day too.

D—DISCOVER

Mindfulness is about discovering more about yourself and the world around you. You become a scientist of your own laboratory—and that laboratory is your body and mind. Notice your habitual patterns of thought. Find out what happens when you meditate every single day for a whole week. Explore what effect fully accepting a so-called negative emotion has on you.

F—FORGIVE

Begin by forgiving yourself for the mistakes you've made. If you've read this far in this book, I have no doubt that you mean well. You want to be a more mindful and conscious person. Accept that as a human you have imperfections. You make mistakes like everyone else on the planet. Condemning yourself just adds to life's burden. Instead, forgive yourself and learn from your mistakes. Then learn to forgive others—not to say what they did was right but for you to stop holding on to grudges. Holding blame is more painful for you than the other person.

U—URGE SURF

This is an unusual one, but you'll find it helpful. Urge surfing is the act of noticing when you have an urge to do something and deciding to just watch that urge rise up and fall instead of fulfilling your desire. This is used in addiction treatment, but in our modern society with the temptations of excessive sweet and fatty food, 24/7 entertainment, cell phones, e-mails, the Internet, and more, we are constantly being tempted. By learning to urge surf, you can notice the urge to check your phone and surf the urge until it passes. Want a second cookie? Feel the urge and see if you can train your brain to sit through it.

L—LOOK AFTER YOURSELF

You may be giving of yourself too much. Constantly helping others without taking time for rest and renewal will drain you. Then you can't help anyone. Looking after yourself with sufficient sleep, exercise, pursuing interests, socializing, having some fun, and meditating are all necessary for human functioning; they are not luxuries.

Finding Ongoing Support

Mindfulness is a popular topic, and there are many resources available to support your efforts, including books about applying mindfulness to specific issues, other guided meditations, local mindfulness meditation groups, mindfulness-based therapists and coaches, online courses and groups, and mindfulness retreats. For a full list, see the Resources in the back of the book.

Week 8 FAQs

This last session is an opportunity to explore any lingering questions that you may have.

Q: **What if I can't stick to my meditation as I've planned to do?**

A: If you think you won't be able to stick to your plan, adjust it. Reduce the time you'll meditate or seek the support of a local weekly meditation group. Or even an online group of meditators could work for you. Give it a try and reassess things in 3 months.

Q: **I didn't really feel I got much benefit from this course. Should I continue?**

A: That's entirely up to you. Just remember that the benefits of mindfulness are subtle and hard to notice at first. I'd suggest, if you're willing, that you practice for a few more months on a daily basis. But it's your choice, of course.

> "Yesterday I looked outside and saw the most beautiful rainbow! Before learning mindfulness, I wouldn't have given it a second glance. Mindfulness has made my life worth living once again. Life is not just clouds and rain. There's also sunshine and rainbows if you look carefully."

Q: **I missed quite a few weeks of the course. Shall I start again?**

A: Yes, you can start again. There's absolutely no harm in that. In fact, practicing an 8-week mindfulness course regularly is a great way to give yourself some structure if you struggle to plan your own time.

Q: **What if I want to do a longer course of mindfulness?**

A: You could do this 8-week course for 8 months. Do each practice for a month rather than a week. I've done that before and found I gained all sorts of new discoveries and insights about myself.

Q: **Even after doing this mindfulness course, I'm still feeling really stressed—my heart is beating fast and I'm always feeling overheated and tense. I can't sleep properly. What shall I do?**

A: Go and see your doctor first. He or she will be able to assess your symptoms properly. Then you'll know if you're suffering from excessive stress or some other condition, or perhaps both. A health professional should be able to point you to other resources or professionals who can help you. If not, find a different doctor or health professional. Your health is a number-one priority.

Home Experiments for the Rest of Your Life

As I mentioned earlier, Week 8 is the rest of your life, so this week's home experiments could be a very long list! But instead, let's keep it simple for this week, and then the following week you can use the plan you've created in your journal using the exercises from today.

1. **Meditation.** Find some time every day to do one meditation of your choice. It could last from 1 minute to 45 minutes—it's up to you.
2. **Mindful living.** Engage in everyday mindfulness—seek to bring your attention back to the present moment whenever and wherever you remember to do so, no matter what you're doing.
3. **Mindful booster.** Choose any mindful booster that you enjoyed working with from the last 7 weeks on this course. One easy choice is simply to spend a few moments every day thinking about and writing what you're grateful for and why.

PRACTICE: Closing Meditation

This is the final meditation to end this particular course. Let the practice signify the start of a new adventure in your life. A new chapter. One in which cultivating greater awareness and self-compassion lies at the heart of your being.

1. Sit or lie down in a posture that feels comfortable for you. Allow your eyes to close gently.

2. Take three deep, full, conscious breaths and then allow your breath to find its own natural rhythm. Feel each precious in- and out-breath.

3. Notice that it's your body breathing by itself rather than you *doing* the breathing. Let your body breathe by itself and be a watcher, an observer of the experience for a few minutes.

4. Open up your awareness to your whole body—feel your body expanding and contracting with each breath. Hold the bodily sensations within awareness.

5. Reflect on all the effort you've taken to meditate over the last 7 weeks. All the moments where you've tried to be mindful. Acknowledge that effort. Be proud of that effort. To get this far, no matter how much meditation you actually did, is admirable. These practices oppose much of what modern culture worships, so congratulate yourself for what you have done so far, rather than berating yourself for what you haven't done.

6. When you're ready, practice some loving-kindness meditation. Begin with yourself if that's okay with you. Use these words, or any other words you prefer:

> "May I be happy. May I be healthy.
> May I be free of suffering."

Allow the words to drop into your heart, not just your head, if you can.

7. Now bring all your friends and family together to mind, including yourself. Use the words:

> "May we be happy. May we be healthy.
> May we be free from suffering."

8. Now consider all the people who practice mindfulness or meditation of some sort, just as you are.

> "May we all be happy. May we all be healthy.
> May we all be free from suffering."

9. Bring all living beings to mind. Plants and trees. All humans and land animals. Fishes in the sea and birds in the air.

> "May we all be happy, healthy, and free
> from suffering."

10. As you bring this meditation to a close, remember that you are

not alone in your meditation—at any time, millions of people are practicing meditation all over the world right now, to manage their stress, to open their hearts, or to create greater peace both within themselves and in the world at large. Dedicate this meditation equally to yourself and all those other people around the world, wishing to be happy and free of their suffering. You are just as worthy of happiness as anyone else in the world.

11. When you're ready, bring the meditation to a close.

VARIATION: Some people like to light a candle or have some flowers or attractive stones placed in front of them when they do this closing meditation, so it feels like a ceremony, signifying the start of a more mindful way of living.

(TIP) You can use this meditation to help you bring a sense of closure to any significant journey or process in your life. The loving-kindness practice in this meditation is particularly good for soothing difficult emotions in your heart and building resilience to future stressors.

Final Words

Thank you for taking this journey into mindfulness together with me. I'm deeply honored that you shared this life-affirming process with me and hope our paths cross in person one day.

Remember, however bad your past has been or however bleak your future may appear, you are not alone. You *can* find relief in the present moment. Take life moment by moment, mindful breath by mindful breath. Joy, peace, and clarity really are accessible to you. I wish you all the very best.

THIRTEEN

Mindful Stretching and Yoga

> *Our bodies are our gardens, to the which our wills are gardeners.*
>
> —WILLIAM SHAKESPEARE

MOVING OR stretching your body can be an enjoyable way of cultivating mindfulness. The stimulus you receive from your body as you begin to gently stretch offers lots of sensations for you to focus your awareness on. For many people, this makes it easier to stay attentive in the present moment and feel centered, grounded, and united with their body.

There are many ways to stretch in a mindful way. The most popular disciplines are probably yoga, tai chi, and qigong. Although yoga is offered in this book, you can practice any approach that appeals to you.

What Is Mindful Yoga?

The word *yoga* means "to join" or "to unite." Yoga is about uniting mind and body. Most people associate yoga with a range of physical postures designed to build flexibility and perhaps promote relaxation or fitness, but yoga is traditionally about developing mindfulness.

The yoga in the MBSR program is not about physical exercise. The focus is far more on the mindful awareness of the various postures you adopt and the transition from one posture to another. You can focus on:

- Your physical sensations from moment to moment, within your body.
- Your breathing.
- How your mind starts to think about other issues and bringing your attention back.

- Your emotions within your physical body.
- Your relationship to the process of stretching. For example, the judgments that pop into your head, your emotional reactions as you hold a pose, your desire to shy away from pushing yourself into a stretch.
- Noticing and letting go of comparison, competition, and judging yourself if you practice yoga with others. Noticing and letting go of the desire to "do," to progress and be able to do certain poses.

If you are uncomfortable practicing yoga because of your religious beliefs, feel free to consider it mindful stretching instead. And use whatever stretches you feel comfortable with—not necessarily yoga postures. This program does not need to be associated with any religion and wishes the process to be accessible to all, whatever your background or physical ability.

Gentle warning: Please remember to check with your doctor before engaging in any physical postures outlined in this book, especially if you have a health condition. If you do have a health condition, you're best advised to work together with a trained and experienced professional instructor who can adapt the movements specifically for you.

> "I had a real resistance to the idea of doing yoga. But when I thought of it as mindful stretching, it seemed much more possible—even I can do a bit of stretching!"

In such a case, consider visualizing yourself in each posture for an equal amount of time as you'd do the real stretch—the imagery will activate the neurons in your brain associated with the stretch, and there's evidence from several studies to

---

Research Corner:
Be Mindful of Your Posture and Feel Great!

Posture can have a direct effect on how you feel. If you're feeling low, simply try sitting up straight, walking upright, and avoiding slouching. It may help reduce your stress by making you feel more in control. And the science seems to agree.

A study published in 2009 in the *European Journal of Social Psychology* by Briñol, Petty, and Wagner asked half of a group to sit slumped and the other half to sit up straight. The people who were sitting up straight had significantly higher levels of self-confidence and belief in themselves compared to those who were slouched. So make sure you stand and sit up straight, especially at your next interview or date!

suggest those muscles will actually strengthen too. This only works if you do the imagery regularly (several times a week for at least several weeks) rather than just once or twice. And the more vivid you can make the imagery, the more effective the outcome seems to be.

Yoga as a Mindful Practice: Being Present in Your Body

Yoga is a superb way to mindfully train yourself to live in the present. And sometimes, when you practice yoga in a mindful way, you may experience a state of flow. Flow is a state of mind in which you are so focused that you notice only what you're engaged in—in this case, yoga. Being aware of your breathing together with your body can often help create this mindful flow state. You forget about your shopping list or the gardening you need to do. You even forget one aspect of living that you're so used to noticing—your sense of self. Your attention is wholly in the moment. You usually also forget about time, as your awareness is so fully present.

This flow state is something you may experience often, sometimes, or never. The most important point is not to try to get into any particular state. Simply be mindful, pay attention with curiosity and openness, and see what happens.

Trees can teach you a lot about yoga and stress reduction. Notice the way trees cope with the wind. As the wind buffets a tree, the branches move and the leaves dance around. They are not stiff or fixed. The top of the tree seems to move the most. But the base of the tree remains fixed and grounded to the earth. The base of the tree is almost completely still. (See the drawing on page 284.)

Yoga is similar. You gently stretch your arms and legs after being buffeted by the stress of the day. But the idea of mindful yoga is that you stay rooted in awareness—just as the tree would topple over without its roots, even though they are invisible. So awareness is your root. And the longer you practice being aware in the present, the deeper your roots and the less likely you are to topple with the stressors you face.

Here are a few tips to consider before you try the yoga practice:

- **Yoga is not about how far you can stretch.** Do you classify the best tree as the one that bends the most? Of course not. In the same way, yoga is not about how flexible you are. The idea is you begin with where you are. Even if after years of yoga practice you were just as flexible as you were when you started, it wouldn't matter—that's not the

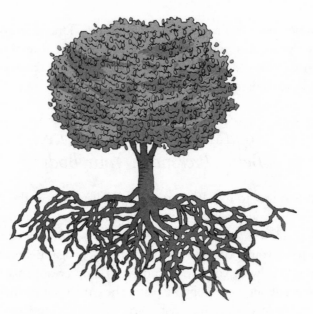

goal. What matters is the level of mindful awareness you brought to the experience.

- **The key to mindful yoga is resting your attention on your breath and bodily sensations.** That's the secret. Just pay attention to your breathing and body. Your mind will wander to thoughts. Those thoughts include judgment, memories, interpretations, ideas, plans, and more. When you notice this happening, acknowledge and bring your attention back to your breathing and your bodily sensations. There's no need to ban thinking. Just notice, smile, and glide your attention back.

- **Yoga is not a competition.** Competition is about comparison and judgment and striving with effort to achieve a goal—comparing yourself to others or to your past achievements. Competition can generate a great deal of motivation, but not usually a reduction in stress, which is what this book is about. You are not good enough now, and you want to be better. So where is your attention? Your attention is on where you want to be, not where you are. And so you are not living in the present. Mindful yoga is about letting go of striving for a goal and just simply being present.

Use your breath like a thread to weave mindfulness into your yoga practice. You can then observe how a posture changes your breath. One posture may deepen your breath, while another may make your breathing more shallow. Holding postures will also affect your breathing—you can watch this with curiosity.

Each time you enter a posture in yoga is an opportunity to discover something new: to discover the relationship between your body, thoughts, and emotions; to discover which muscles feel tight, your emotional reaction to any intense sensations, and the thoughts that arise in your mind.

If you're an experienced yoga practitioner, you may want to do more advanced postures, and that's fine. But even the most adept practitioners can learn and grow from practicing each of these postures with mindfulness and as if for the first time, with a sense of freshness and playfulness.

Want a Yoga Class?

In addition to learning basic yoga from this book, you may like to try a class. The benefit of joining a class is that the teacher can show you how to do the poses and correct any mistakes you may be making. Being with others in the class and making friends can be an additional stress reliever.

Here are a few tips for finding an appropriate teacher:

- Is the teacher experienced? How many years? Is the teacher qualified?
- Is the yoga class for relaxation and stress reduction or some other goal? Hatha yoga is often more slow and mindful, but almost any yoga can be taught in a mindful way.
- Is the class suitable for beginners or not?
- If you have a specific health condition, check that the teacher can adjust the class appropriately.

Experiencing Yoga (and Life) with Playfulness

Playfulness is a mindful attitude. One enjoyable way to practice yoga is to bring an attitude of playfulness. See if you can find some joy in the various poses. If you can, great. If you have difficulty feeling joy for anything, that's okay. You may have been through a significant amount of stress, which prevents you being able to feel happiness at the moment. In this case, bring as much mindful awareness to the poses as you can and hold a very gentle and subtle smile on your face. Research suggests the nerves in your facial muscles will begin sending signals to your brain, helping to gently lift your mood.

As a child you were able to find joy in the simplest activities. That inner child has not gone away—you're always able to tap into that resource. Experiment with bringing a childlike curiosity to your own body as you practice some yoga today and see what happens.

Most experts agree that play is helpful to reduce not only children's stress but adults' stress too. Playfulness indicates that a marriage will last longer. Playfulness is identified, by psychologists studying happiness, as one of the 24 top most important human strengths. If you have a hobby or activity that you do every day or week just for fun, you're more likely to do that activity with mindful awareness and therefore reduce your stress too.

I personally had an inner resistance to yoga practice when I learned it in a class. The first time I really enjoyed practicing yoga was actually when I was training to teach mindfulness with Jon Kabat-Zinn, developer of MBSR. He was teaching trainee mindfulness teachers and encouraged us all to bring a spirit of playfulness to the whole yoga practice. He invited us to imagine we were like babies, lying in our cots, stretching our bodies as if for the first time. This made the process far more enjoyable and effortless for me.

PRACTICE: Mini-Mindful Yoga Sequence

Audio track 9: 10 minutes.

Standing Mountain Yoga Pose

Begin by standing up straight. Allow your big toes to touch, but your heels can be slightly apart. If you find it hard to balance, you can have

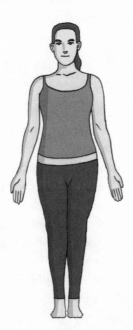

your feet a few inches apart. Firm your thigh muscles so they lift your kneecaps, but try to keep your abdomen relaxed. Feel a gentle sense of yourself lengthening. Rotate your pelvis so your tailbone is tucked in and your pubis is moving up toward your navel. Press your shoulders back and down, opening your chest. Ensure your head is balanced centrally on your neck. Feel each in-breath and each out-breath.

Upward Salute

On your next inhale, raise your arms outward and stretch toward the sky. Feel the sensations in your arms and shoulders as you stretch. Hold your palms parallel to each other, above your head. Tip your head back slowly and gently—there's no need to force your head back too far. Extend your tailbone toward the floor. Keep breathing with mindful awareness in this posture for a few breaths. Breathe out and sweep your arms outward and begin to bend downward. As you bend down, move on to the next posture, the standing forward bend.

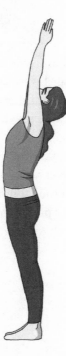

Forward Bend Pose

As you exhale, contract your thigh muscles. Keeping your legs slightly bent to protect your back, bend forward from your hips, not your waist.

Feel your breath releasing and the sensation in your legs and back as you go down. Just notice how far you can go.

Relax your head and neck and allow your arms to be limp. Keep feeling your breathing and let yourself relax on each out breath. If you feel uncomfortable, you can bend your knees a little more.

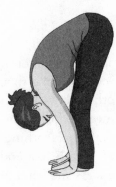

Cobra Pose

Now lie on your front and stretch your legs back, with the top of your feet on the floor. Place your hands on the floor, under your shoulders. Keep your elbows in toward your body. Gently push the front of your feet and thighs into the floor. Be mindful of your breathing.

On your next in-breath, slowly push your hands down to lift your body upward. Rise only to a height at which your pelvis and legs stay in connection with the floor. Continue to feel each in- and out-breath. Push your shoulders back. See if you can allow the bend to be distributed throughout your whole spine. You need to hold this pose for only about 10 seconds. Then, on your next exhalation, slowly lower yourself back to the floor. You can repeat this sequence two more times if that feels okay.

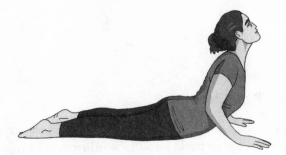

TIP The key is not to overdo the back bend. To test whether you're overdoing it, lift your hands off the mat for a moment and see if you can hold the posture. Remember, you're focusing on using mindful awareness to reduce your stress, not put excessive physical tension in your back.

Cat Pose

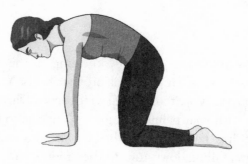

Cow Pose

1. Come up on your hands and knees on the floor. Keep your knees underneath your hips. Make sure your shoulders, elbows, and wrists are in a straight line. Keep your head positioned so that it's neither looking up nor drooping down. Instead, simply gaze at the floor. This is a neutral, tabletop posture. As you exhale, arch your back toward the ceiling. You can allow your head to go down, but you don't need to force your chin to your chest. As you inhale, return to the neutral tabletop pose and go into the cow pose. Feel your breath expanding both your belly and your lower back—this pose gives you a unique opportunity to try to feel your breath in your back.
2. Lift your sitting bones and chest upward, which allows your stomach to move downward. At the same time, lift your head so you're looking straight ahead.

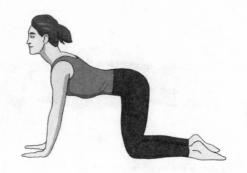

3. On your next exhale, go back to the cat pose.

4. Repeat this in rhythm with your breathing 10–20 times if that feels okay.

(TIP) You need to be careful to protect your neck by keeping your shoulders down, away from your ears.

Child's Pose

To get into child's pose, begin by kneeling on the floor. Allow your big toes to touch and then gently sit on your heels. You can then separate your knees so they are roughly hip width apart. Place your arms alongside your torso with your palms facing up. Continue to feel the sensation of your breathing. Each time you breathe, have a sense of your shoulders relaxing and falling down toward the ground. This is a resting posture, so you don't need to strain. After a minute or so, on your next exhalation, slowly rise up from the pose.

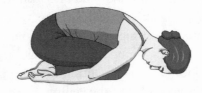

(TIP) To make the pose more challenging and deepen the stretch, stretch your arms forward in front of you, while drawing your shoulders back and down.

Corpse Pose

Finish your yoga practice today with corpse pose as described in Chapter 4.

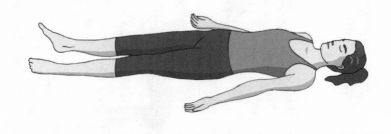

PRACTICE: Full Mindful Yoga Sequence

Audio track 10: 30 minutes.

If you're doing the full MBSR course using this book, begin with the mini sequence described above. Then go straight into the poses in this section, which take another 20 minutes.

1. Continuing to be in corpse pose, on your next in-breath, move your arms directly above your head and stretch your heels in the other direction. Breathe in and out and notice all the sensations throughout your body as you do this. On your next out-breath, bring your arms back to your sides. Take a few mindful breaths.

2. Now place your feet on the floor so your knees point toward the ceiling. Draw both your knees toward your chest and hold on to your knees. Gently rock from side to side, massaging the muscles in your back. If you want, you can raise your head toward your knees. You can also try some gentle circling movements on your back. Practice this for a few breaths and then stretch your legs back out. Notice how your body feels now.

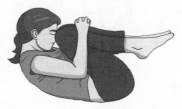

3. Draw in your left knee with your hands, not forcing it too much toward yourself. If you wish to go deeper into the stretch, bring your head toward your knee as far as it can comfortably go. Feel the sensation in the stretch. Then after a few breaths, stretch your left leg out. Repeat this process with your right leg.

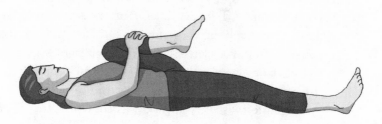

4. Lie down on your back again with your arms by your sides. Notice how your body feels now, just being with your body and your breathing.

5. Raise your knees so your feet are as close as possible to your buttocks. Place a blanket under your shoulders if you wish. As you breathe out, push down on your feet so you raise your lower back off the floor. Keep your knees over your heels. There's lots of space above and below your abdomen to breathe—notice this. When it's right for you, come back down again as slowly as possible. Then stretch your legs out and be aware of how your body feels as you lie down.

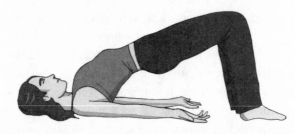

6. Lie down on your mat again. Bring your knees up to your chest and hug them if you can. Feel a few breaths mindfully. Then gently rock from side to side or up or down to massage your back. If you wish, bring your head toward your knees on your next out-breath. Then when you're ready, stretch your legs back out again.

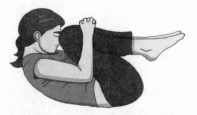

7. As you lie on your back, place your arms perpendicular to your body, forming a T shape. Raise your knees with your feet on the floor. Then tighten your tummy muscles and let your knees come down to your left side, slowly. Your right knee may be able to follow or may not. Just go as far as you comfortably can. At the same time, turn your head toward the right so you're creating a gentle twist in your body, as shown in the diagram. On

> "Being quite fat and inflexible, I never thought I had a hope in hell of achieving anything with the yoga. But somehow the mindfulness increased my confidence and I began to stretch and exercise my body for the first time in years."

each out-breath, see if you can relax into the posture so gravity can gradually deepen the twist. No need to force anything. When you're ready, tighten your tummy muscles again as you raise your knees and roll them over to the right side and look toward the left, feeling your breathing and naturally allowing gravity to pull your legs down into the mat, quite naturally. After a few breaths, tighten your stomach muscles and come back into the center and then stretch your legs out.

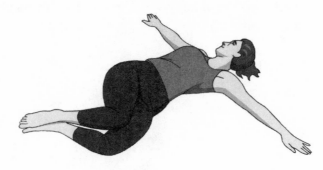

8. Now slowly stand up and come into mountain pose. Take a few deep, conscious breaths. Allow your breathing to find its natural rhythm. Feel the sensations throughout your body as you stand for a minute or so.

9. **Pointing upward.** As you breathe in, lift your arms above you, touching your hands together, with your fingers pointing toward

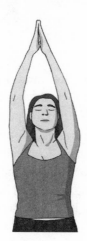

the ceiling. When you're ready, lower your arms so you're form-ing a cross. Hold this posture for a few breaths. Now bring your arms back down again into mountain pose.

10. **Picking a fruit.** Lift your left arm up so it's stretching above your head, leaving your right arm by your side. Stretch your left arm as far as you can, as if you're trying to pick a fruit just beyond your reach. To increase the stretch, stand on tiptoes on your right foot. Feel the stretch in the left side of your body and notice whether your right side is tensing unnecessarily. When you're ready, slowly lower your left arm, past the horizontal and feel the sensation in your arm—notice your breathing as you go back into mountain pose. Then repeat this process with your right arm.

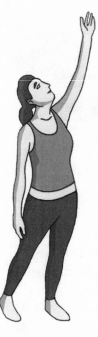

11. **Bending to the left and right.** Now raise both your arms together, up through the horizontal position and into a vertical position, so your arms are pointing up past your ears toward the ceiling or touching each other. Feel the stretch in your arms. When you're ready, slowly bend to the right. Your bend is from the hip, and your body will bend to maintain balance. Hold this position, keeping your head between your arms. Keep breathing rather than holding your breath. Find your edge—not too far, but feeling a stretch. Then, after a few breaths, bring both your

arms above your head again. Repeat this procedure, bending to your left.

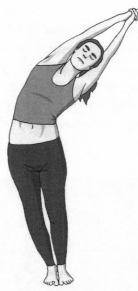

12. **Mountain pose.** On your next out-breath, allow your arms to come back down again into the mountain pose. Stand balanced and solid. Notice what it is like to be in this standing posture after doing those stretches. Bring your awareness back to the rhythm of your own breathing.

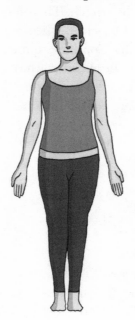

13. **Shoulder rolls.** When you're ready, try a few shoulder rolls. Begin by pushing both your shoulders forward, keeping your chest in the same position. Then let your shoulders drop down. Now move your shoulders back as if you're trying to touch your right and left shoulders behind you. Then lift up your shoulders so they can almost touch your ears. Then just let your shoulders drop down. Repeat this process for a few cycles. Then, after a few rolls, go in the opposite direction—up, back, down, and forward. Return to mountain pose when you feel you've done enough.

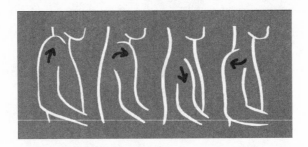

14. **Head rolls.** Allow your head to drop gently to your right side. Let the weight of your head allow the stretch of your head so your right ear is moving toward your right shoulder. Now roll your head around so your chin is dropping down toward your chest. Feel the stretch. Then rotate around so your left ear is over your left shoulder. Then move back around to your right shoulder again. Continue to rotate slowly in this way. Let the weight of your head control the depth of the stretch. After a few cycles, go around in the other direction. When you're ready, come back into mountain pose.

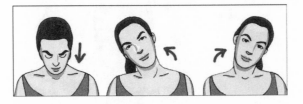

15. **Balancing pose.** With this awareness of your center of balance, lift your arms to your sides so they form a horizontal line with your fingertips pointing outward. You may find it helpful to find

a point on the floor or wall to focus your attention on. Form a cross with your body and shift your balance to your right foot. As you move all your weight to your right foot, lift your left foot slowly off the floor and point it to your left. You may need to keep bringing your left leg down, or you may find a point of balance with your left leg up. Then, when you're ready, bring your left leg back down again. When you're ready, repeat this process on the other side, with most of your weight on your left and your right leg raised. Then, when you've finished, bring your leg and arms down slowly at the same time and adopt the mountain pose once again.

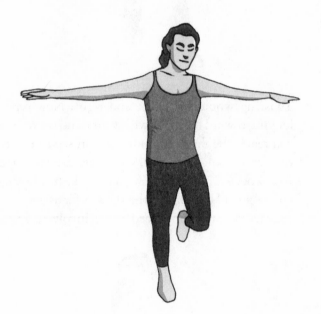

16. In **mountain pose,** notice any physical release that may be happening. The sense of relief at the end of the last pose, the change in your breathing rate or depth, any tingling sensations in your body. Stay in this posture until you're ready and willing to move on.

17. **Looking left and right.** Place both your hands on your hips, just moving your head to the right. Begin with just your eyes looking toward your right and then your chin. Go as far as you can without pain. Relax your shoulders if they've become tense. When you're ready, move your head back to facing forward. And then repeat to the left, beginning with your eyes and then your head. Then return to center.

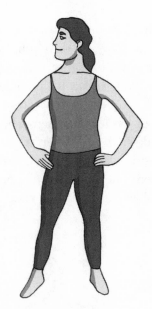

18. **Twisting whole body left and right.** Now repeat the process looking toward the right with your hand on your hips. But when you reach the farthest point you can see to the right, continue the twist from your waist. Continue the twist right down into your knees and ankles. So your neck, head, waist, knees, and ankles are all twisting to the right as far as you can. Notice what muscles do and don't need to be involved. Explore your own

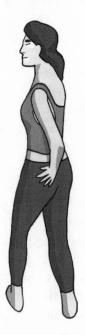

limit, your edge. When you're ready, come back into the central position and rotate and twist to the left as far as you can. Then release your arms back into the mountain pose.

19. **Mountain pose.** Finish in mountain pose. Notice what it feels like. Be aware of your whole body from the top of your head to the tips of your toes. Notice any sense of warmth or coolness.

20. **Acknowledge** the time you've taken for yourself and that this subtle process will have a positive effect, like a ripple, in both your day and your whole life.

Reflection

How did you respond to the mindful yoga? What thoughts, feelings, and bodily sensations did you notice in particular? What positive effects do you think this sequence would have on you if you practiced it on a regular basis? Note your observations in your journal.

Resources

Your Mindfulness Audio

This book comes with a set of free guided mindfulness meditations that you can download. Visit *www.guilford.com/alidina-materials* to download it onto your computer or mobile device.

Finding an MBSR Teacher Near You

INTERNATIONAL

University of Massachusetts Medical School (UMMS)—Center for Mindfulness in Medicine, Health Care, and Society
www.umassmed.edu/cfm

To find an MBSR teacher near you, you can begin by contacting UMMS's Center for Mindfulness. They will probably have a list on their website in the near future too.

UNITED KINGDOM

Be Mindful
http://bemindful.co.uk/

This has a list of the latest MBSR courses, as well as teachers, mainly located in the United Kingdom. Again, not comprehensive, but worth a look.

INTERNATIONAL

Many online lists are not always up to date. The best way to find a mindfulness teacher in your area may be to use a search engine like Google. For example, if you want to find a mindfulness teacher in San Francisco or Holborn, just search "mindfulness holborn"/"mindfulness san francisco" or "mbsr holborn"/"mbsr san francisco." You could also try searching "mbct holborn"/"mbct san francisco."

Many MBCT (mindfulness-based cognitive therapy) teachers are able to teach MBSR too. And the programs are quite similar.

With this approach, you need to find out what credentials the teacher has and judge whether he or she seems sufficiently qualified and has the necessary experience. Ask them who they trained with and how long they've been teaching mindfulness.

Online Mindfulness Courses

www.shamashalidina.com

I offer a free 21-day e-course introduction to mindfulness when you sign up on the website. It's also a way of keeping in touch with my work.

www.livemindfulonline.com

This is my popular video-based 8-week mindfulness course with downloadable audio meditations.

www.bemindfulonline.com

This website has a 4-week mindfulness course.

Recommended Websites

Mindful
www.mindful.org

A well-written and well-designed website and monthly magazine with all the latest news and tips in the world of mindfulness. Some excellent articles from the best teachers are available here.

Mindfulnet
www.mindfulnet.org

A website with a wealth of resources, links, and information on mindfulness for stress and mindfulness in the workplace.

Greater Good Berkeley Center
http://greatergood.berkeley.edu

This is a great website with evidence-based resources on cultivating gratitude, altruism, compassion, empathy, forgiveness, happiness, and mindfulness. All these qualities have been linked to greater resilience against stress.

Action for Happiness

www.actionforhappiness.org

A great nonprofit organization with a wealth of well-designed and -researched resources to help you to raise your own happiness and help others to be happier.

Dalai Lama

www.dalailama.com/messages/compassion

This is a fantastic short piece written by His Holiness the Dalai Lama on "Compassion and the Individual." I'm sure you'll find inspiring ideas on managing your stress and increasing your happiness in that article.

American Institute of Stress

www.stress.org

The American Institute of Stress is a nonprofit that imparts information on stress reduction, stress in the workplace, effects of stress, and various other stress-related topics.

Finding a Mindfulness Retreat

I run secular mindfulness retreats once or twice a year—contact me for details. You could also try searching for mindfulness retreats in your area; with the increase in mindfulness teachers around the world, there may be one nearby.

The following websites list lots of established centers that offer mindfulness retreats. The websites often have links to other recommended centers that may be more convenient for you.

Gaia House—Devon, United Kingdom

http://gaiahouse.co.uk

Spirit Rock—Woodacre, California

www.spiritrock.org

Insight Meditation Society—Barre, Massachusetts

www.dharma.org

Plum Village—Southern France

http://plumvillage.org

Deer Park Monastery

http://deerparkmonastery.org

Books

MINDFULNESS AND WELL-BEING

Alidina, Shamash. (2010). *Mindfulness for dummies.* Chichester, West Sussex, UK: Wiley.

Brahm, Ajahn. (2010). *Opening the door of your heart: And other Buddhist tales of happiness* (new ed.). Sydney: Read How You Want.

Cutler, Howard C., & Dalai Lama. (1998). *The art of happiness: A handbook for living.* New York: Riverhead Books.

Hanh, Thich Nhat. (1991). *Peace is every step: The path of mindfulness in everyday life.* New York: Bantam Books.

Kornfield, Jack. (2002). *A path with heart: The classic guide through the perils and promises of spiritual life.* London: Rider.

Ricard, Matthieu. (2006). *Happiness: A guide to developing life's most important skill.* New York: Little, Brown.

MINDFULNESS FOR STRESS

Kabat-Zinn, Jon. (2013). *Full catastrophe living: Using the wisdom of your body and mind to face stress, pain, and illness* (rev. ed.). New York: Bantam Books.

Williams, Mark, & Danny Penman. (2011). *Mindfulness: An eight-week plan for finding peace in a frantic world.* New York: Piatkus.

SELF-COMPASSION

Germer, Christopher K. (2009). *The mindful path to self-compassion: Freeing yourself from destructive thoughts and emotions.* New York: Guilford Press.

Neff, Kristin. (2013). *Self-compassion.* London: Hodder & Stoughton.

Salzberg, Sharon. (1995). *Loving-kindness: The revolutionary art of happiness.* Boston: Shambhala.

STRESS MANAGEMENT

Alidina, Shamash. (2012). *Relaxation for dummies.* Chichester, UK: Wiley.

Charlesworth, Edward A., & Ronald G. Nathan. (2001). *Stress management: A comprehensive guide to wellness.* New York: Atheneum.

Davis, Martha, Elizabeth Robbins Eshelman, & Matthew McKay. (2008). *The relaxation and stress reduction workbook.* Oakland, CA: New Harbinger.

MINDFUL MOVEMENT

Boccio, Frank. (2004). *Mindfulness yoga: The awakened union of breath, body and mind.* Boston: Wisdom.

Hanh, Thich Nhat, & Wietske Vriezen. (2008). *Mindful movements: Ten exercises for well-being*. New York: Parallax Press.

If You Need Help Urgently

If you're feeling distressed and don't know where to turn to for whatever reason, or are contemplating suicide, contact the Befrienders Worldwide. They are a network of 169 emotional support centers in 29 countries. They link to centers that provide essential support to people in crisis for free. They will listen without judging you.

www.befrienders.org

References

References are listed in the order in which the material cited appears in the book so you can get more detailed information from the source as you read the chapters if you like.

Chapter 1

Perkins, A. (1994). Saving money by reducing stress. *Harvard Business Review, 72*(6), 12.

How stress can cause depression. (n.d.). *ScienceNordic.com*. Retrieved from *http://sciencenordic.com/how-stress-can-cause-depression*.

Csikszentmihalyi, M. (1990). *Flow: The psychology of optimal experience*. New York: Harper & Row.

Lieberman, M. D. (2010). Dispositional mindfulness and depressive symptomatology: Correlations with limbic and self-referential neural activity during rest. *Emotion, 10*(1), 12–24.

DeLongis, A., Folkman, S., & Lazarus, R. S. (1988). The impact of daily stress on health and mood: Psychological and social resources as mediators. *Journal of Personality and Social Psychology, 54*(3), 486–495.

Goeders, N. E. (2003). The impact of stress on addiction. *European Neuropsychopharmacology, 13*(6), 435–441.

Killingsworth, M. A., & Gilbert, D. T. (2010). A wandering mind is an unhappy mind. *Science, 330*(6006), 932.

Parswani, M. J., Sharma, M. P., & Iyengar, S. S. (2013). Mindfulness-based stress reduction program in coronary heart disease: A randomized control trial. *International Journal of Yoga, 6*(2), 111–117.

Gregg, J. A., Callaghan, G. M., Hayes, S. C., & Glenn-Lawson, J. L. (2007). Improving diabetes self-management through acceptance, mindfulness, and values: A randomized controlled trial. *Journal of Consulting and Clinical Psychology, 75*(2), 336–343.

Deyo, M., Wilson, K. A., Ong, J., & Koopman, C. (2009). Mindfulness and rumination: Does mindfulness training lead to reductions in the ruminative thinking associated with depression? *Journal of Science and Healing, 5*(5), 265–271.

Creswell, J. D., Myers, H. F., Cole, S. W., & Irwin, M. R. (2009). Mindfulness meditation training effects on CD4+ T lymphocytes in HIV-1 infected adults: A small randomized controlled trial. *Brain, Behavior, and Immunity, 23*(2), 184–188.

Davidson, R. J. (2003). Alterations in brain and immune function produced by mindfulness meditation. *Psychosomatic Medicine, 65*(4), 564–570.

Zeidan, F., Martucci, K. T., Kraft, R. A., Gordon, N. S., McHaffie, J. G., & Coghill, R. C. (2011). Brain mechanisms supporting the modulation of pain by mindfulness meditation. *Journal of Neuroscience, 31*(14), 5540–5548.

Howell, A. J., Digdon, N. L., & Buro, K. (2010). Mindfulness predicts sleep-related self-regulation and well-being. *Personality and Individual Differences, 48*(4), 419–424.

Farb, N. A., Anderson, A. K., Mayberg, H., Bean, J., McKeon, D., & Segal, Z. V. (2010). Minding one's emotions: Mindfulness training alters the neural expression of sadness [correction to Farb et al. (2010)]. *Emotion, 10*(2), 215–215.

Jha, A. P., Stanley, E. A., Kiyonaga, A., Wong, L., & Gelfand, L. (2010). Examining the protective effects of mindfulness training on working memory capacity and affective experience. *Emotion, 10*(1), 54–64.

Moore, A., & Malinowski, P. (2009). Meditation, mindfulness and cognitive flexibility. *Consciousness and Cognition, 18*(1), 176–186.

Carmody, J., & Baer, R. (2008). Relationships between mindfulness practice and levels of mindfulness, medical and psychological symptoms and well-being in a mindfulness-based stress reduction program. *Journal of Behavioral Medicine, 31*(1), 23–33.

Creswell, J. D., Irwin, M. R., Burklund, L. J., Lieberman, M. D., Arevalo, J. M., Ma, J., et al. (2012). Mindfulness-based stress reduction training reduces loneliness and pro-inflammatory gene expression in older adults: A small randomized controlled trial. *Brain, Behavior, and Immunity, 26*(7), 1095–1101.

Vøllestad, J., Nielsen, M. B., & Nielsen, G. H. (2012). Mindfulness- and acceptance-based interventions for anxiety disorders: A systematic review and meta-analysis. *British Journal of Clinical Psychology, 51*(3), 239–260.

Borders, A., Earleywine, M., & Jajodia, A. (2010). Could mindfulness decrease anger, hostility, and aggression by decreasing rumination? *Aggressive Behavior, 36*(1), 28–44.

Barnes, S., Brown, K. W., Krusemark, E., Campbell, W. K., & Rogge, R. D. (2007). The role of mindfulness in romantic relationship satisfaction and responses to relationship stress. *Journal of Marital and Family Therapy, 33*(4), 482–500.

Lucas, M. (2012). *Rewire your brain for love: Creating vibrant relationships using the science of mindfulness.* Carlsbad, CA: Hay House.

Chapter 3

Ullrich, P. M., & Lutgendorf, S. K. (2002). Journaling about stressful events: Effects of cognitive processing and emotional expression. *Annals of Behavioral Medicine, 24*(3), 244–250.

Chapter 4

Surawy, C., Roberts, J., & Silver, A. (2005). The effect of mindfulness training on mood and measures of fatigue, activity, and quality of life in patients with chronic fatigue syndrome on a hospital waiting list: A series of exploratory studies. *Behavioural and Cognitive Psychotherapy, 33*(1), 103–109.

Bjergegaard, M., & Milne, J. (2013). *Winning without losing: 66 strategies for succeeding in business while living a happy and balanced life.* London: Profile.

Shapiro, S. L., Carlson, L. E., Astin, J. A., & Freedman, B. (2006). Mechanisms of mindfulness. *Journal of Clinical Psychology, 62*, 373–386.

Jain, S., Shapiro, S. L., Swanick, S., Roesch, S. C., Mills, P. J., Bell, I., et al. (2007). A randomized controlled trial of mindfulness meditation versus relaxation training: Effects on distress, positive states of mind, rumination, and distraction. *Annals of Behavioral Medicine, 33*(1), 11–21.

Chapter 5

Rozin, P., & Royzman, E. B. (2001). Negativity bias, negativity dominance, and contagion. *Personality and Social Psychology Review, 5*(4), 296–320.

Joseph, S. (2011). *What doesn't kill us: The new psychology of post-traumatic growth.* New York: Basic Books.

Rosenkranz, M. A., Davidson, R. J., MacCoon, D. G., Sheridan, J. F., Kalin, N. H., & Lutz, A. (2013). A comparison of mindfulness-based stress reduction and an active control in modulation of neurogenic inflammation. *Brain, Behavior, and Immunity, 27*(1), 174–184.

Chapter 6

Killingsworth, M. A., & Gilbert, D. T. (2010). A wandering mind is an unhappy mind. *Science, 330*(6006), 932.

Mark, G. J., Voida, S., & Cardello, A. V. (2012). A pace not dictated by electrons: An empirical study of work without email. In *Proceedings of the SIGCHI Conference on Human Factors in Computing Systems* (CHI '12). New York: 555–564.

Ophir, E., Nass, C., & Anthony, D. W. (2009). Cognitive control in media multitaskers. *Proceedings of the National Academy of Sciences USA, 106*, 15583–15587.

Farb, N. A. S., Segal, Z. V., Mayberg, H., Bean, J., McKeon, D., Fatima, Z., et al.

(2007). Attending to the present: Mindfulness meditation reveals distinct neural modes of self-reference. *Social Cognitive and Affective Neuroscience, 2*(4), 313–322.

Chapter 7

Cannon, W. B. (1939). *The wisdom of the body.* New York: Norton.

Selye, H. (1956). *The stress of life.* New York: McGraw-Hill.

Keller, A., Litzelman, K., Wisk, L. E., Maddox, T., Cheng, E. R., Creswell, P. D., et al. (2011). Does the perception that stress affects health matter? The association with health and mortality. *Health Psychology, 104*(4), 716–733.

Could stress be good for you? Research that suggests it has benefits (TED blog). (n.d.). Retrieved from *http://bit.ly/stresscanbegood.*

Aschbacher, K., O'Donovan, A., Wolkowitz, O. M., Dhabhar, F. S., Su, Y., & Epel, E. (2013). Good stress, bad stress, and oxidative stress: Insights from anticipatory cortisol reactivity. *Psychoneuroendocrinology, 38*(9), 1698–1708.

Holmes, T. H., & Rahe, R. H. (1967). The social readjustment rating scale. *Journal of Psychosomatic Research, 11*(2), 213–218.

A new stress paradigm for women. (n.d.). Retrieved from *www.apa.org/monitor/julaug00/stress.aspx.*

Pace, T., Negi, L., Adame, D., Cole, S., Sivilli, T., Brown, T., et al. (2009). Effect of compassion meditation on neuroendocrine, innate immune and behavioral responses to psychosocial stress. *Psychoneuroendocrinology, 34*(1), 87–98.

Chapter 8

The science of mindfulness meditation. (n.d.). Retrieved from *http://psychcentral.com/news/2007/06/22/the-science-of-mindfulness-meditation/910.html.*

Can mindfulness increase our resilience to stress? [video file]. (n.d.). Retrieved from *www.youtube.com/watch?v=ALjFlyb-VLw.*

Creswell, J. D., Way, B. M., Eisenberger, N. I., & Lieberman, M. D. (2007). Neural correlates of dispositional mindfulness during affect labeling. *Psychosomatic Medicine, 69*(6), 560–565.

Chapter 9

Cuddy, A. (n.d.). *Your body language shapes who you are.* Retrieved from *www.ted.com/talks/amy_cuddy_your_body_language_shapes_who_you_are.*

Carney, D. R., Cuddy, A. J., Yap, A. J. (2010). Power posing: Brief nonverbal displays affect neuroendocrine levels and risk tolerance. *Psychological Science, 21*(10), 1363–1368.

Pennebaker, J. W., Kiecolt-Glaser, J. K., & Glaser, R. (1988). Disclosure of traumas and immune function: Health implications for psychotherapy. *Journal of Consulting and Clinical Psychology, 56,* 239–245.

Smyth, J. M., Stone, A. A., Hurewitz, A., & Kaell, A. (1999). Effects of writing about stressful experiences on symptom reduction in patients with asthma or rheumatoid arthritis. *Journal of the American Medical Association, 281,* 1304–1309.

Open up! Writing about trauma reduces stress, aids immunity. (n.d.). Retrieved from *www.apa.org/research/action/writing.aspx.*

Chapman, S. G. (2012). *The five keys to mindful communication: Using deep listening and mindful speech to strengthen relationships, heal conflicts, and accomplish your goals.* Boston: Shambhala.

Hanh, T. (1975). *The miracle of mindfulness: An introduction to the practice of meditation.* Boston: Beacon Press.

Chapter 10

Neff, K. (2013). *Self compassion.* London: Hodder & Stoughton.

Kok, B. E., & Fredrickson, B. L. (2010). Upward spirals of the heart: Autonomic flexibility, as indexed by vagal tone, reciprocally and prospectively predicts positive emotions and social connectedness. *Biological Psychology,* 432–436.

Lanxon, N. (2012, July 12). *Compassion over empathy could help prevent emotional burnout.* Retrieved from *www.wired.co.uk/news/archive/2012-07/12/tania-singer-compassion-burnout.*

Ricard, M. (2013, October 9). *Empathy fatigue.* Retrieved from *www.matthieuricard.org/en/blog/posts/empathy-fatigue-2.*

Klimecki, O. M., Leiberg, S., Ricard, M., & Singer, T. (2014). Differential pattern of functional brain plasticity after compassion and empathy training. *Social Cognitive and Affective Neuroscience, 9*(6), 873–879.

Klimecki, O., Ricard, M., & Singer, T. (2013). Empathy versus compassion: Lessons from 1st and 3rd person methods. In T. Singer & M. Bolz (Eds.), *Compassion: Bridging practice and science* (pp. 272–287). Retrieved from *www.compassion-training.org.*

Chapter 11

What you need to know about willpower: The psychological science of self-control. (n.d.). Retrieved from *www.apa.org/helpcenter/willpower.aspx.*

Does self-compassion or criticism motivate self-improvement? (n.d.). Retrieved from *www.psychologytoday.com/blog/the-science-willpower/201206/does-self-compassion-or-criticism-motivate-self-improvement* .

Boehm, J. K., & Kubzansky, L. D. (2012). The heart's content: The association between positive psychological well-being and cardiovascular health. *Psychological Bulletin, 138*(4), 655–691.

Aked, J., Marks, N., Cordon, C., & Thompson, S. (2009). *Five ways to well-being:*

A report presented to the Foresight Project on communicating the evidence base for improving people's well-being. London: NEF.

Oman, D., Thoresen, C. E., & McMahon, K. (1999). Volunteerism and mortality among the community-dwelling elderly. *Journal of Health Psychology, 4*(3), 301–316.

Chapter 13

Brinol, P., Petty, R. E., & Wagner, B. (2009). Body posture effects on self-evaluation: A self-validation approach. *European Journal of Social Psychology, 39,* 1053–1064.

Index

About the Author

Shamash Alidina has been helping people to manage stress using mindfulness for more than 14 years. He is the author of the bestselling *Mindfulness for Dummies*. Based in London, he teaches mindfulness internationally to health professionals, executive coaches, and the public. He also offers mindfulness teacher training programs online. His website is *www.shamashalidina.com*.

List of Audio Tracks

TRACK 1.   Two-Minute Mindfulness Exercise—2 minutes (Chapter 1)

TRACK 2.   Opening Awareness Meditation—10 minutes (Chapter 4)

TRACK 3.   Uncovering Your Intention: Mindful Ocean Visualization—10 minutes (Chapter 4)

TRACK 4.   Mindfully Eating an Apple—10 minutes (Chapter 4)

TRACK 5.   Mindful Belly Breathing—10 minutes (Chapter 4)

TRACK 6.   Mini-Body Scan Meditation—10 minutes (Chapter 4)

TRACK 7.   Full Body Scan Meditation—30 minutes (Chapter 4)

TRACK 8.   Mindful Pause Meditation—2 minutes (Chapter 5)

TRACK 9.   Mini-Mindful Yoga—10 minutes (Chapter 6)

TRACK 10. Full Mindful Yoga—30 minutes (Chapter 6)

TRACK 11. Mindful Walking—10 minutes

TRACK 12. Mindfulness of Breath Meditation—10 minutes (Chapter 6)

TRACK 13. Mini-Mindfulness of Breath and Body Meditation—10 minutes (Chapter 7)

TRACK 14. Full Mindfulness of Breath and Body Meditation—20 minutes (Chapter 7)

TRACK 15. Mini-Expanding Awareness Meditation—10 minutes (Chapter 8)

TRACK 16. Full Expanding Awareness Meditation—30 minutes
(Chapter 8)

TRACK 17. Responding to Stress Meditation—10 minutes (Chapter 9)

TRACK 18. Mountain Meditation—20 minutes (Chapter 10)

TRACK 19. Lake Meditation—20 minutes (Chapter 10)

TRACK 20. Loving-Kindness Meditation—30 minutes (Chapter 10)

TRACK 21. Silence with a Bell in Between—10 minutes total

TRACK 22. Silence with Bells Every 5 Minutes—30 minutes total

TRACK 23. Silence with Bells Every 10 Minutes—30 minutes total

TRACK 24. Silence with Bells Every 15 Minutes—45 minutes total